My Own Technique Of Eating
For Health

My Own Technique Of Eating For Health

by J. I. Rodale

RODALE PRESS, INC.
Book Division
Emmaus, Penna. 18049

STANDARD BOOK NUMBER 0-87857-006-3

LIBRARY OF CONGRESS CATALOG CARD NUMBER 71-81786

COPYRIGHT MCMLXIX BY J. I. RODALE

ALL RIGHTS RESERVED

PRINTED IN U.S.A.

PB-37

THIRD PRINTING—MAY 1971

1. No Milk

In 1940 I first came in contact with the idea that milk was not all it was cracked up to be. At the time, I was publishing a magazine called *True Health Stories,* and in it I included a story, "Cutting Out Milk Cured my Arthritis." It was by Theo. F. Huber, and I will reproduce a part of it:

"Years ago owing to the continual cracking noise in my joints, I became aware of a tendency toward arthritis. As time passed the trouble became worse and I finally consulted a physician.

"He medicated me according to his best ability, but his treatment failed to give me any relief. Later I came to the conclusion that medicine could afford no cure so I stopped doctoring entirely.

"The disease finally became serious to the extent that my neck would stiffen at times and remain rigid for days. Not knowing which way to turn and getting very eager to do something for myself, I decided to try a change of climate.

"I had been living in New York State all my life. It seemed as if the severe winters and damp springs always aggravated my condition, so I determined to try the warmth and dryness of Southern California. One year out there helped me somewhat, at least the progress of the disease seemed to have been arrested but I had not been helped to the degree I had hoped for. So I left California for Florida to continue my experiment. The tropical warmth of Florida was too damp for me and aggravated my condition.

"I was now sure that I could never obtain complete relief through climate changes and that my condition could only be benefited through a radical change in my diet. Accordingly I read everything I could find regarding arthritis and its treatment through diet.

"One so-called authority recommended foods rich in Vitamin B. Another emphasized the virtues of fresh fruit juices. Others recommended a complete abstinence from all flesh or animal foods and concentrated starches like cereals and potatoes, all of which I tried out with variable results, allowing sufficient time in each instance for the experiment.

"My diet for years had consisted mostly of milk, cottage cheese, whole grain products, fruits and vegetables. Milk products were so highly recommended and advertised as the best food for health that it never occurred to me to question the claims of the advertisers. However, a time did come when I did question their claims and the challenge came in a most unexpected way.

"A series of business reverses had forced me from a desk in a Wall Street bank to a placer gold mine in California. Due to my inaccessible location in the mines, I was unable to contact a regular supply of fresh milk so that for the first time in 30 years I was actually forced to go without it. Result: the very first month following my abstinence I noticed a distinct change for the better in my condition. As time went on the improvement continued and became so pronounced that I was rendered entirely free from every trace of arthritis by the end of the 7th month.

"However, to really prove and satisfy myself that milk had been the cause of my trouble, I decided to return to using it, inasmuch as I was now able again to obtain a regular supply.

"To make a long story short, within six weeks all my old arthritis symptoms had reappeared. Every joint in my body ached when moved just as they had done previously. Especially my neck, which at times would crack as loud as the snap of the fingers. The return experiment had proved beyond a question of doubt that milk and cottage cheese were the causes of all my trouble, so I abandoned the use of them and have never returned to them since."

Later this story was reprinted in another magazine I published, *Fact Digest,* and we added the following letter to it:

"Some four months or so ago I read in the columns of *True Health Stories* an article written by a sufferer of arthritis who told of testing everything he did and ate, to try to find out the cause of his troubles. The last thing he tested was the drinking of milk, of which he was a generous user. Immediately his arthritis disappeared, after years of afflicting him.

"When I read the article I questioned it, but was interested for I had been a victim of arthritis for about ten years. At the same time I suffered from ulcers of the stomach and the doctor urged me to use milk generously as he regarded it as the best stomach medicine. I did not realize that the more milk I used the more painful was my arthritis. I spent hundreds upon hundreds of dollars taking treatment from regular M.D.'s, osteopaths, Swedish movement treatments, etc. One was as great a 'flop' as the others so far as relief was concerned. So as a last resort, after reading the article, I cut milk out of my diet entirely. Within a week or two my arthritis disappeared and seems to

[3]

have entirely cut my acquaintance, for which I am grateful.

H. L. Aldrich,
New York, N. Y."

*   *   *   *

These reports started my interest in a diet free of milk. Although they are just reports by individuals who were not scientists, in later years I found many medical researches which showed that milk is not the ideal food for adults that many people thought it was.

Over the years I have accumulated medical data proving that milk-drinking is one of the greatest blunders in our modern diet. In this case I played the role of a compiler, an aspect of medical science which is greatly neglected.

Today hundreds of thousands of persons are not consuming milk and other dairy products because of what they have been reading in *Prevention*.

The July, 1955, issue was entirely devoted to the negative qualities of milk. The first article was the following:

I don't drink milk, and am not ashamed to admit it. I have been away from milk drinking now for over 5 years and as yet there have been no signs of any deficiencies or repercussions of any kind. So far my body has taken no reprisals against me. At first there was a feeling of anxious uncertainty. Would lightning and thunder figuratively come and destroy me for such sacrilege? Not only has nothing of the kind happened, but I am going my merry way, thriving healthfully without milk, full of buoyant energy and with the confident feeling that (pardon the grammar) me and the cow (that is, its liquid white portion) have parted ways forever.

[4]

Now, from whence comes my calcium if I do not get it from milk? I get it from *bone meal!* If there had been no bone meal substitute, there could have been trouble unless in expert fashion the rest of the diet had been tailored to make up for that calcium deficit.

My wife hasn't drunk milk or eaten any cheese since she was weaned. For some mysterious reason she developed a deep-rooted aversion to milk and its whole family of related products. Yet today she is as hard as a rock.

In thinking back about milk I recalled a visit I once made many years ago to a farming school where a herd of cows was kept. This was a school, mind you, not a private farm or dairy. When I went into the place where the cows were being milked I immediately experienced a suffocating tightness. I will admit that the ventilation in the barn was poor. The next morning I had the most beautiful case of septic sore throat of my entire life. As you read various articles about milk you will come across some statements about septic sore throat being transmitted through milk, in spite of pasteurization.

Looking back at all these facts I still hesitated to take up my cudgels in print against milk. For years I thought and thought about it, debating whether or not we should tell our readers what we knew against milk drinking, but it seemed too revolutionary a thing to do. Such a sacred attitude had been built up toward milk that it had become more than a fetish. Down through the ages it had become a powerful symbol. It had grown into a magic belief, a refuge, a sort of sacred fountain from which one drank and imbibed eternal youth. How could we snatch away this source of comfort from our friends?

But my conscience could not remain quiet. When

[5]

I saw people breaking every rule of health and then resorting to milk as if it would quench all this error, I became aroused. When I realized how many persons are needlessly suffering through an overconsumption of milk, I came to a decision. I would do it regardless of consequences. I would cast the data I had upon the waters. If it comes as a shock to some, I hope that they will study the matter most thoroughly, possibly experimenting a little before they make up their mind.

I will say one thing most positively—if you think that milk, as it is produced under modern conditions, will be an appreciable factor in giving you health, I must tell you that you are not basing your belief on reality. Today's emasculated product is unfit for human consumption, not to mention the needs of the calf itself for whom the milk was intended. Poor thing! The modern calf is not growing up into a healthy cow.

This is proven by the increasing use of the antibiotic drugs given to cows. No one can tell me that this doesn't affect the cow's meat and its milk in some detrimental way. I have before me several strange circulars issued by the Tarkio Molasses Feed Co. of Kansas City. One of them, dated March 22, 1955, and addressed to "Dear Cattle Feeder," says, regarding the stilbestrol drug approved a few months ago by the U. S. Food and Drug Administration, that it causes meat to go "soft" and not to age properly, and that their company did not intend to put any stilbestrol into its cattle feed. The other circular is a letter from the Williams Meat Co. of Kansas City, one of the outstanding meat provisioners of our country today, which furnishes the best of meat for many large fancy restaurants. Here is what Mr. Williams of that company said in a letter to the Tarkio Molasses Feed Co. on March 14, 1955: "As you know we specialize in prime quality

[6]

meats, making Kansas City meats nationally famous. For some reason in recent months, the texture of the meat is exceptionally soft and not responding to proper aging. Are feeders experimenting too much with drugs?"

Much of this sort of wonder drug feeding is "happening" to cows and I wonder what it will do to the milk? At any rate, the whole thing is so unpredictable that one will never know at what moment Bossy will be given another "wonder" treatment, without administrators waiting the necessary time for laboratory checking of dangers.

A great part of milk's popularity is due to the propaganda of the milk interests. Powerfully organized, they send their tons of literature to the schools, P.T.A.'s and other places where it will do the most good. I recall an experience I had seven or eight years ago which threw some light on this activity. When we started the Soil and Health Foundation I had some correspondence with a professor in a dental college who wished to know whether I could run an experiment on our farm, feeding two groups of mice—one with food raised with chemical fertilizers, the other with food raised by the organic method. Then he came to the farm for further discussions. He advised that the experiment would be financed by a big milk foundation, but when he said that milk had to be one item of food for each group of mice, and when I expressed a few negative thoughts about milk, he left, never to return. I received no more letters from him.

Much of our opinion regarding the healing quality of milk stems from this endless stream of propaganda— a torrent of advertising costing hundreds of millions of dollars. We are bombarded by it at every turn, through the newspapers, radio and television, until milk has become crowned with a halo. But it is a halo purchased with dollars, and therefore I do not feel guilty when I tarnish it a little.

There is no question that milk has a delightful, satisfying taste—so has strawberry shortcake with ice cream. However, one cannot live by taste alone if one wishes to live a long, healthy life, although there is nothing wrong with the taste of apples, carrots, and roast beef.

My diet consists of meat, fish, eggs, vegetables (mostly raw, some cooked) and a lot of fruit. I do not eat anything that has gone through a factory, and to me milk is a highly factoryized thing—not only because of pasteurization but also because a high production factory has been made out of the cow's udders. I eat no bread or cakes, and no soups, because I am on a reducing diet. But my diet is a very satisfying one with the aid of some black coffee, which I am forced to take because of a heart condition that I am holding in wonderful subduedness with the aid of vitamin E. I take a great many different natural vitamins, plus bone meal.

I am on a low salt, no sugar diet, and because of this and my general diet, my blood pressure is like that of a newborn babe—120 over 70. Before I began all this I had a very high blood pressure.

You can point to some persons who are heavy milk drinkers and yet who are perfectly healthy, but it is possible that it is the way they are built. Perhaps they have wider arteries than the average person and a more tuned-up set of glands. It is the way they were born, due to their heritage. Those are the people who smoke and drink and live to over 80. But you and I may not be in that class.

Some think that babies cannot get along without milk. Liquefied meat used with a formula containing about the same amount of protein, carbohydrate, fat and mineral content of cow's milk proved valuable in a recent study of infants who were allergic to cow's milk. An article in *California Medicine* for October 19, 1954, describes the work of several doctors who gave lamb meat with vegetable oil and potato starch or tapioca flour as a starch. Later, as the need for solid food arose, they gave additional strained meats, pureed vegetables and fruits. Over 100 infants and children who had eczema, bronchial asthma and digestive disturbances were given the meat formula for more than three months. In no instance was there any loss of weight, or anemia. In most cases there was a rise in the red coloring matter of the blood, and improvement in whatever the disorder had been.

Dr. Henry C. Sherman, Columbia University's outstanding nutritional authority, has said that in studying the nutritional needs of man you cannot deal exclusively in terms of known chemical factors. You have to include "natural articles of food," he says, to "ensure adequate supplies of any possible factors which may not yet have been identified and listed in chemical terms. We must give emphasis to those foods which, as the 'natural wholes' to which our species is nutritionally adjusted by its evolutionary history, will furnish us, along with the known essentials, any unknown factors which may also be essential to our nutrition." Could Dr. Sherman have been referring to seeds? They certainly are "natural wholes."

Two other nutritional experts, Burr and Burr, have shown that a diet may be complete in all essentials, including minerals, vitamins, proteins, etc., but if it lacks the unsaturated fatty acids, which are obtained chiefly from seeds, nutritional deficiency will result. Of course, the average eater is bound to get some seeds in his diet such as peas, beans, nuts, wheat, corn, etc., but if he is conscious of their importance he will find ways to add more of them to his total food intake.

2. Sugar

IN MY MAGAZINE *True Health Stories* I found an article (May, 1940) entitled "Cut Out Sugar—Cured a Nervous Breakdown," by Clara E. Smith. It was my first encounter with the idea that sugar could be harmful to the human body.

I will give you the article in its entirety:

*   *   *   *

It was in 1920 when I had a nervous breakdown. I had taught music for ten years, so steadily, that I went "to pieces"—as we say. I went to my physician often and one day he said to me: "No, I won't give you a drop of medicine. You just want to put a lash on a worn out horse—well I won't give you the lash. Nerves! nerves! nerves!" he called after me.

Another doctor told me, very politely in suave tones, you "may live five years."

Another doctor gave me ten years to inhabit this earth.

There was yet one more M.D. to consult, and he said, "You are headed for the insane asylum. It is rather hard too. That is a nice boy you have there." My little son was with me.

Each physician knew I was a piano teacher and

made that the goat for my extreme nervousness. For financial reasons I had to stay at my work, though at times I could only teach part of the pupils that came.

After the last verdict the doctors had given, I went for a walk to fight things out in my mind.

It was winter. The ground was frozen hard. I turned from the town and walked along the road, by empty fields, and all was as gloomy as my thoughts.

I stumbled along. I had no desire to return home. I was just in despair. What was the use of anything? Hadn't I tried through my college days—worked overtime to make my life a success? Where were the dreams I had for later years? Stumbling over a raised portion of ground, I caught hold of a top rail of a fence, and looking up I faced a sky like gold—turning into crimson and more gold, and fleecy clouds like gold lace, floating through the bluest sky I had ever seen. I took hold of the fence rail with a strong grip.

"I do not believe a word any of the doctors say. I will be strong and live," I thought, and I knew no one doomed to die could really walk so many miles and be lifted to such heights at the vision of a sunset while clinging to a fence rail on a winter day.

When I reached home and had entered the house, I sank into a chair. The old fear and trembling had returned. I wanted no food. I agreed that the doctors were right, and I didn't care anyway.

An hour later, my son's daddy came and laid a new magazine near me. I paid no heed until the lights came on and with the brightness my spirits rose, and I looked through the article of which I want to tell you. It was in MacFadden's publication called *Physical Culture*. It dealt with the record of a physician who reached such a physical state that no medical advice could help him, stating it in this way, "They made

[11]

me feel after a consultation much the same as a dog must feel when they tie fire crackers to his tail and tell him to lie down and rest." Out of his abject misery he decided sugar was a cause of nervousness and did without any sugar for three months.

He was cured. I resolved to try the plan, using for the necessary sweets, raisins, honey, and dates. For three months I used no sugar. At the end of that time I called on my first doctor again. I was entirely composed and my hands were steady. The doctor peered over his glasses and said, "What have you done to yourself? You look like a new person. Want medicine today?" "No," I replied. "I have decided not to put a lash on a worn out horse."

"You didn't use sugar . . .? Well you need it for energy and warmth—but I do remember you were a wreck when you went out of here. No sugar— Humph!" He tossed his papers about on his desk.

Since that three months' trial, I have had no recurrence of that dreadful time. Besides the prohibitive sweet I would not allow dark thoughts to enter my mind, and tried to keep something colorful about me. Twenty years longer, I have continued my teaching.

*   *   *   *

3. Some Facts About Sugar

IN READING the *New York Times* the other day (October 24, 1951) I came across a news item regarding a round-table discussion at the 20th Annual Meeting of the American Academy of Pediatrics at Toronto, Canada. Among other erudite subjects, they took up the question of fleas and insects. They stated that flea bite is a condition well known on the West Coast, but is now becoming more common in the East. Doctors were advised, they said, to consider it seriously as a possible cause of certain skin troubles. They overlooked the fact that there are certain researches which absolutely indicate that where the body is well nourished (which means then that the skin is well nourished), fleas will not find such a habitation palatable to them. A flea is an insect that thrives on a skin that is filthy or diseased, and in most cases such diseases cannot be seen with the naked eye. There is a condition known as a subclinical form of scurvy with which more than 60 per cent of our population is now afflicted.

In experiments with dogs, where certain doses of vitamin C were given, the fleas left for other parts. No flea would inhabit the skin of a dog who did not have a vitamin C deficiency.

This is merely a prelude to the main theme. At this meeting, in a further discussion of insect bites, but not specifically fleas, Dr. Earl D. Osborne of Buffalo referred to a certain piece of research which indicated that Vitamin B_1 given to individuals in quantity, by mouth, seemed to act as an insect repellent. This is where sugar comes in. But first let me give you my story.

About five years ago, I decided to cut all artificial sugars out of my diet. This was on the advice of Dr. Melvin E. Page of St. Petersburg, Florida. Dr. Page has a laboratory in which he checks the blood of patients. He has found that normally the blood of a person who is healthy and does not eat artificial sugars, has a certain relationship between its calcium and

[13]

phosphorus. He has found it is two and one-half to one, or two and one-half times as much calcium as phosphorus. But in all his experience, he finds this ratio grossly distorted in the blood of patients who are sugar-consumers. When that was explained to me, I immediately realized that I wanted to have my blood as healthy as possible, and began to eliminate severely all these artificial sugars. However, I could eat fruits and such things as honey and molasses in moderation.

That summer I noticed that I was practically immune to mosquito bites. When all others were complaining about being bitten, I was not. And when I discussed this matter with an aunt of mine who has diabetes, and who also has to forego artificial sugars, she said she has had the same experience. She does not get bitten by mosquitoes.

Now here is the most interesting thing about this whole subject. The doctor mentioned earlier, who gave vitamin B_1 to individuals to act as an insect repellent, was working within the scope of a program that cuts out sugar. This is how it works:

I have since found out that artificial sugars use up vitamin B_1 in the body. This would seem to indicate that people who are using artificial sugars in their diet are not only distorting the calcium-phosphorus ratio in their blood, but are also destroying vitamin B_1. This loss can lead to many serious conditions.

I might state that alcohol also uses up the vitamin B_1 in the body. People who drink habitually, that is, take liquor every day, will usually suffer from a severe vitamin B_1 deficiency. That is why in the treatment of alcoholism, tremendous doses of vitamin B_1 are given to these unfortunates.

I had a very interesting experience recently in meeting with a former aviation pilot who was active in

[14]

World War II. He told me that he used to suffer from blackouts. They would take only a few seconds, but in a plane that would be a very serious and dangerous thing. The doctors cured him by giving him vitamin B_1. This would seem to indicate that airplane pilots should not eat sweet foods such as ice creams, pies, pastries and others that contain artificial sugars, including cola drinks. Chances are, if this pilot had been on a diet that eliminated artificial sugars, he probably would not have suffered from these blackouts caused by vitamin B_1 deficiency, and cured by taking vitamin B_1.

It is amazing how a mosquito can detect that the blood is not to its liking. In other words, a mosquito is practically a censor, determining whether there is too much calcium or phosphorus for his taste. Probably he has a sense of smell that can detect an odor from blood not properly constituted for him. I should not want to go around with my blood out of whack, however slight such a distortion should be. The body should be running like a Swiss watch mechanism. Can you picture a Swiss watch with something only slightly out of whack? That would not do. An article called "Down the Pike" by E. S. Bayard, from the *Pennsylvania Farmer*, May 28, 1949, throws additional light on the subject of diet and mosquitoes:

"I have had some chance to observe the effects of diet, or at least what I was told were such effects. The people of Peru are the smallest I have ever seen. And in the market at Lima the portions of meat sold are the smallest I have seen anywhere on three continents. But these two things don't prove anything—they may be merely coincident facts. Many years ago in Western Canada the late Herbert Quick and I went to a church event where ice cream and other good things were served. The air was full of mosquitoes and there was a smudge fire in each corner of the yard where the good things were supplied. Mr. Quick and I ate with two Indian women who admired his books. Not a mosquito was on the arms or face of either lady. I was told that this was because they ate no sugar—but that may not be the real reason.

When white people are going into the tropics where mosquitoes may be carrying some kind of serious disease, I think it would be a good idea for them to go into training first and for a long period preceding the trip, take all the artificial sugars out of the diet and possibly add a little vitamin B_1 besides. If this fact had been known in the Spanish-American war, many lives might have been saved!

4. Mosquito Bites

In the December, 1953, issue of *Prevention* I made some observations about mosquitoes. A reader had written in describing an experience he had: "A friend of mine was working in northern Canada where there was a settlement of Indians. It was during the black fly season and it was quite evident that the flies were concentrating on jabbing me, while the Indian chief who sat nearby was entirely free of them. My astonished friend asked why. The chief's reply was, 'One month before the black fly season all Indians naturally know enough to leave all sugars from their diet.' " We civilized Americans, with all our knowledge of chemistry, have not figured out a number of basic facts about nutrition that are well known to primitive people.

[16]

When some New York friends visited the farm, we were talking about the mosquito scare and sleeping sickness in Florida, and I related to them that since I eat no sugar, the mosquitoes never bother me. Other persons, at the same time, are almost eaten up by them.

One of the visitors told me that this was true as far as he was concerned, because he was very careful about his sugar consumption. He said that occasionally there are mosquitoes in his apartment. They trouble his sugar-eating roommate, but not him.

In my book *The Healthy Hunzas,* which is about a race of people located in the northwest tip of India, I have shown how disease-free they are. It is interesting to note that they absolutely do not have available any of the artificial sugars of civilization.

I want to close with an interesting experience that I recently had. I know a biochemist in Philadelphia who is helping people by testing their blood specifically for vitamin deficiency and prescribing the lacking vitamins. I have seen three cases in which this physician helped immensely. A few weeks ago I took a friend to see this doctor and went along personally to see how it was done. This patient was suffering from hay fever, and the doctor took some of his blood and tested it right before my eyes on a spectroscope. The blood of this patient showed all kinds of deficiencies. Then the doctor looked at me with a peculiar gleam in his eye and said "Look here, Rodale, you are supposed to be eating food raised organically and you are always talking about your wonderful health. Now I've got you here, let me take some of your blood and test it."

I said, "Sure, go ahead."

When he tested some of my blood, he looked at me and said: "Rodale, this is the best blood I have seen in the year and a half that I have been doing this kind

[17]

of work, and bear in mind that I have been testing blood of healthy people, as well as sick ones, for many persons come here for routine checkups."

But the one thing he particularly showed me was my calcium-phosphorus relationship. He said he rarely comes across a case where it is as close to the two and one-half to one as mine was. My calcium was 10.00 and my phosphorus was 4.575 milligrams. The patient that I brought along had calcium 8.895 and phosphorus 4.620.

This shows what clean living will do.

5. The Cornaro Story

At this point I am rambling through some old files of magazines I published from about 1935 to 1943. There was *Fact Digest, You Can't Eat That,* and *True Health Stories.* As I read, I wince occasionally as I come across articles representing health viewpoints with which I violently disagree today.

But in this pleasant browse I found an article which should be made part of this book, as it aided me in my climb to better health. I will present it here. It is entitled: "Cornaro Ate Sanely—and Lived Long" (March, 1940, *True Health Stories*).

Louis Cornaro was an Italian nobleman who, some 400 years ago, lived such a riotous youth that the doctors gave him up for an incurable invalid by the time he had reached the age of forty. He was weak. His digestion was impaired. His resistance to infection

[18]

was lowered. He had continual aches and pains. The physicians told him his only chance of living a few years longer lay in his immediately changing his mode of living. Cornaro realized the seriousness of his condition and took their advice to heart. He changed his eating and drinking habits—*and he lived in peace and health to the ripe old age of* 98 *years!*

Here's how he did it:

He observed a strict regimen in regard to moderate exercise, sleeping and eating. He exercised, slept and ate at regular times—and he ate sparingly. He never overloaded his stomach. He always rose from the table with an appetite. "In this manner," he wrote, "I conformed to the proverb, which says that a man, to consult his health, must check his appetite."

Within a year these living habits made Cornaro a fairly healthy man. Once he had regained his health he did not return to his former dissipations. Realizing the preciousness of his newfound physical comfort, he continued to eat and drink sparingly.

For good health and long life, wrote Cornaro in his book *How to Live to Be a Hundred,* people should not "eat a greater quantity of any kind of food, even of that which agrees with them, than their stomachs can easily digest; the same is to be understood of drink."

Cornaro clearly realized that his long life was primarily made possible by his changed habits of living. At the age of 83 he put his formula for longevity in writing. At the age of 86 he penned a second treatise on living long. Again and again throughout his writing he echoes that warning—don't overeat if you want to enjoy a long, happy life.

Of persons who "eat till their stomachs are overburdened with much food," wrote Cornaro, "I never knew any person, who led that kind of life to be very

[19]

old. All these old men I have been speaking of would live long, if, as they advanced in years, they lessened the quantity of their food, and ate oftener, but little at a time."

Further, says Cornaro, "nor am I apt to be drowsy after meals; the food I take being in too small a quantity to send up any fumes to the brain. O, how advantageous it is to a man to eat but little! Accordingly, I, who know it, eat but just enough to keep body and soul together. . . . O, what a difference there is between a regular and an irregular life! One gives longevity and health, the other produces disease and untimely deaths."

These words were written some four hundred years ago. Their good counsel and plain warning is as sound today as it was then. Far too many people in this modern era habitually eat and drink to the point of indulgence—and far too many die before reaching the advanced age possible for all persons, barring accident, to enjoy.

*　　*　　*　　*

We later published a translation of Cornaro's book, which we titled *How to Live to Be* 100 (it is now out of print, but can be seen at public libraries). There are many interesting details of his method in it. But I would like to show his fondness of meats by quoting that he liked "some broth with an egg in it, or such other good kinds of soup or spoon meat. Of flesh meat, I eat veal, kid and mutton. I eat poultry of every kind. I eat partridges and other birds, such as thrushes. I likewise eat fish."

He also stated that he ate some bread. It, of course, was the Italian bread made of nothing more than flour and water, but when one considers the small amount of his daily food intake, and the fact that he rode horseback into his eighties, one can see that he compensated for the small amount of bread he consumed. However, had he eaten no bread at all, he might have lived even longer.

Cornaro said that the total weight of all the food he ate was only 12 ounces per day—¾ of a pound. Some people eat a pound of wheat stuffs a day. Cornaro's wine consumption was 14 ounces, but when he was about 70 his family and friends became so alarmed at his meager consumption of food that, fearing for his life, they brought pressure to bear and he increased his daily food intake from 12 to 14 ounces, his wine from 14 to 16 ounces.

His reaction: "This increase and irregularity had, in 8 days' time, such an effect upon me, that, from being cheerful and brisk, I began to be peevish and melancholy, so that nothing could please me and I was constantly so strangely disposed that I neither knew what to say to others, nor what to do with myself. On the 12th day I was attacked with a most violent pain in my side, which held up 22 hours, and was succeeded by a terrible fever, which continued 35 days and as many nights, without giving me a moment's respite . . .

"But, God be praised, I recovered merely by my former regular course of life, though then in my 78th year, and in the coldest season of a very cold year."

Cornaro relates how at the age of 70 he was in a coach, "which going at a pretty smart rate, was overset, and in that condition drawn a considerable way by the horses, before means could be found to stop them; whence I received so many shocks and bruises, that I was taken out with my head and all the rest of my body terribly battered, and a dislocated leg and arm.

[21]

"When I was brought home, the family immediately sent for the physicians, who, on their arrival, seeing me in so bad a plight, concluded that within three days I should die; nevertheless, they would try what good two things would do me; one was to bleed me, the other was to purge me; and thereby prevent my humors altering, as they every moment expected, to such a degree, as to ferment greatly, and bring on a high fever.

"But I, on the contrary, who knew, that the sober life I had led for many years past, had so well united, harmonized, and disposed my humors, as not to leave it in their power to ferment to such a degree, refused to be either bled or purged. I just caused my leg and arm to be set, and suffered myself to be rubbed with some oils, which they said were proper on the occasion. Thus, without using any other kind of remedy, I recovered, as I thought I should, without feeling the least alteration in myself, or any other bad effects from the accident; a thing which appeared miraculous even in the eyes of the physicians."

*   *   *   *

Cornaro at first experimented to see what foods agreed with him. He found the following bad: "Very cold wines, as likewise melons and other fruits, salad, fish and pork, tarts (cake), gardenstuff, pastry, and the like . . . by experience I limited the use of such foods and wines, and likewise of ice; in less than a year [this diet] rid me of all disorders which had taken so deep a root in me. I used to be attacked every year with a strange kind of fever, which sometimes brought me to death's door."

At the age of 95 Cornaro wrote a short treatise to acquaint his fellowman with his system, and how it had aided him to live and enjoy a healthy life to so

[22]

advanced an age. At this age he found himself "sound and hearty, content and cheerful." He writes, "All my faculties are as good as ever, and in the highest perfection, my understanding clearer and brighter than ever, my judgment sound, my memory tenacious, my spirits good, and my voice, the first thing which is apt to fail in others, grown so strong and sonorous, that I cannot help chanting out loud my prayers morning and night, instead of whispering and muttering them to myself, as was formerly my custom . . . nor yet can the thoughts of death find room in my mind. Neither can the death of grandchildren and other relations and friends make any impression on me, but for a moment or two, then it is over!"

I would like to reproduce here the beautiful Eulogy of Cornaro, introduced by Antonio Maria Graziani, in his life of Cardinal Commendoni: "This most illustrious man, upon whom the title of 'The Sober' has been so appropriately bestowed, was loved, honored, and reverenced by all who were distinguished by birth or acquirements. People of every class, from the noble to the peasant, were delighted to associate with him, and to listen to his conversation, which was always marked with moderation, amiability, and good sense. Prudence, sagacity, wisdom, and liberality were constant attendants in his train. There was no mansion in Padua, the sight of which inspired such reverence as his; while he, living in a style of princely magnificence, was continually dispensing his favors to all, and, in especial, to the cultivators of the fine arts."

Incidentally Cornaro's mansion in Padua, Italy, is still standing.

One more final thought: Opponents of the organic method of agriculture accuse it of being impractical because the yields would be reduced, and thus there

[23]

would not be enough food to go around. First of all, the organic method increases rather than reduces yields, but even if it did reduce them, it would force the world to eat less, and thus become healthier.

6. Aluminum Cooking Utensils

IN 1942 I first heard that cooking in aluminum utensils could be dangerous to health. The subject was covered in an article printed in our *Fact Digest* (June, 1942), entitled "Poisons Formed by Aluminum Cooking Utensils," by H. J. Force, which had appeared in *Naturopath* magazine. I was so impressed that we immediately got rid of all our pots and pans and began to cook in stainless steel, here and there in glass, and some in enamel.

Here is a digest of the article mentioned:

* * * *

In the 21st edition of the *United States Dispensatory,* published in 1928, under "Alum" on page 109 and under "Uses," we find the following:

"Alum is a powerful astringent with very decided irritant qualities, and when taken internally in sufficient quantities is emetic and purgative, and may even cause gastro-intestinal inflammation. It is widely employed in various conditions in which an astringent or styptic is desired. . . . *When small quantities* of the soluble salts of aluminum are introduced into the circulation they produce a slow form of poisoning characterized by motor palsies and areas of local anesthesia with fatty degeneration in the kidney and liver. The nerve symptoms have been shown by Doellken to be due to anatomical changes in the nerve centers. There are also often symptoms of gastro-intestinal inflammation which is presumably the result of the effort of the glands of the intestinal tract to eliminate the poisoning . . ."

Aluminum chloride compounds will be formed when vegetables are cooked in aluminum to which a small quantity of salt (sodium chloride) has been added. Many natural waters contain quite a little salt. It is evident that when such waters are used when cooking in aluminum, aluminum chloride will be formed.

It has been shown that aluminum compounds precipitate or destroy the pepsin which is the principal ingredient in digestion. Alum is a compound of aluminum, potash, sulphur and oxygen, together with a small portion of water. When vegetables are cooked in aluminum vessels, they often contain such compounds as sulphur, potash or soda, which could easily combine with the aluminum, forming small quantities of alum, also aluminum sulphate.

Many drinking waters throughout the United States are very hard, containing a large portion of sulphur compounds, also potash and soda. In fact, some waters which I have analyzed become alkaline on boiling. As potash and soda very readily dissolve aluminum, forming a compound similar to alum in its composition, it follows that this compound will be formed if aluminum utensils are used for any length of time to cook food products.

Sauerkraut, when cooked in aluminum, will produce aluminum chloride, especially if allowed to stand for some time. Many cases of poisoning, and some deaths, have resulted from sauerkraut being cooked in aluminum.

*   *   *   *

From this statement it is evident that indigestion and constipation could be produced, and that the kidneys and liver could be affected with most serious results.

Here we have the highest authority in the United States telling us of the poisonous effects of aluminum.

When aluminum cooking utensils are used, there is always some aluminum dissolved. The amount will depend upon the kind of water used. At picnics, church suppers and other places where large numbers are served, the foods are often allowed to stand for some time in aluminum. As a result we often read in the newspapers of numbers of people being stricken ill very soon after eating, probably poisoned from the aluminum compounds formed. Death sometimes follows.

People often say they like to use aluminum utensils, as foods do not burn when cooked in such utensils. The reason is that some aluminum is always dissolving, forming hydrogen gas, and so pushing the foods away from the aluminum. The same thing applies to an aluminum griddle. Salt and soda are generally used in the batter, and these increase the solubility of the aluminum.

Large doses of aluminum compounds are often fatal. Small quantities may be taken daily with little or no effect. But sooner or later, indigestion, constipation, Bright's disease or diabetes may develop as a result of the continued use of aluminum ware.

Some claims have been made that aluminum is not soluble when used for general cooking purposes. Statements of this kind are absolutely false, and show the gross ignorance of such writers. There is not a single

[26]

laboratory in the United States that would think of using aluminum vessels for making chemical analyses.

To show the solubility of aluminum, make the following simple test for yourself: Place in a well cleaned and scoured aluminum utensil, one quart of water, a good pinch of salt and a pinch of baking soda, and let boil for one hour, adding water to make up the loss. Then remove from the fire and let stand for 2 or 3 hours, then pour into a glass jar and notice the milky condition caused by aluminum hydroxide. This will settle out in a day or so, but its presence is proof that aluminum is soluble.

From the *Dispensatory* and various *materia medica,* it is apparent that the nation is being poisoned. There never was so much sickness and complaining, never so much stomach disorder, etc. Cancer has jumped from tenth to second place as the cause of death in the last 10 years. Yet at the same time we have more medical knowledge, more doctors, hospitals, radio lectures on health, newspaper articles on how to keep well, etc., yet sickness is still on the increase. There must be a reason.

Aluminum will affect the teeth, as this chemical has an affinity for calcium, and is so stated by dentists who have investigated the action of aluminum on the teeth. It is also possible for the aluminum to affect the calcium in the bones.

Try this test: Put one-half of a can of tomatoes in an aluminum vessel, and the other half in an agate ware vessel. Add the same amount of salt and baking soda to each. Cook and then let stand for 24 hours, then reheat, and note the difference in taste. We would not advise you to eat the tomatoes cooked in the aluminum. Those cooked in the agate will be good eating.

If tomatoes are cooked in a dull-appearing aluminum

[27]

utensil, the acid in the tomatoes will act upon the aluminum, giving it a very clean appearance. The amount of aluminum removed is of course dissolved into the tomatoes.

Most vegetables contain a tiny amount of aluminum, about one part in a million, but in an entirely different form from that which is dissolved when cooking foods in aluminum. The white powder often seen when cooking potatoes in aluminum is aluminum hydroxide, which is harmless.

Remember, the continued use of aluminum wares will finally produce results which will be similar to leaving the foods standing in them for some time. It is the small quantities absorbed from the foods, as *Dispensatory* points out, which may produce indigestion, nervousness, constipation, cancer, etc.

7. Organic Foods Make Us Healthier

AT THIS TIME I would like to reproduce an article from the December, 1945, issue of *Organic Gardening*, showing how we reacted to the eating of organically raised food:

We purchased a farm of 63 acres but I could take no physical part in its operation because of the pressure of business interests. It went along under the handicap of wartime labor shortages and farmhands who were indifferent, independent and inexperienced.

Mistakes in cultural practices were frequent, but one thing we did—we made and spread compost. We used not an ounce of artificial fertilizers or poison sprays.

We fattened steers and raised chickens but had no cows because of the impossibility of building suitable structure during wartime. Every bit of feed for chickens and steers was raised on our own farm organically and it showed in our having very fine, healthy animals. We thus had our own steer and chicken meat and eggs but no milk. The rest of our organic diet was from vegetables out of our own garden, and sunflower seeds. I would say that about 30 per cent of our diet was produced organically.

My seven-year-old daughter, Nina, was chosen by the school nurse as having the finest teeth in her class. About seven or eight years ago the dentist would always find one or two cavities in my teeth every six months. In the last two years he hasn't found any. About two years ago there was a small beginning of one but the dentist, during the wartime pressure of work, decided to wait till the next visit. At the next session he found that it had proceeded no further so he postponed action again. It is now two years and that tiny, open cavity has progressed no further.

I used to get a severe headache every few weeks but in the last year have practically had none. You cannot imagine what a delightful thing it is to be free of dreadful headaches, and not have to take aspirins or bromo seltzers. But my most remarkable benefit is in my practical immunity to colds, for there I had a very gory record. A few years back I had a half dozen severe colds one winter, a practically continuous affair, which seriously interfered with my work. During the winter of 1944 I had two slight colds, of very short duration, but the autumn season of 1945 was the first time in forty years that I did not contract a cold in September when the first cool weather arrived. There is something about a change in the weather that always gave me a cold, but not so this year, and I was exposed several times under severe conditions, wearing thin summer clothes. In the old days that would have meant a sure cold.

I must say also that my mind functions more clearly in the last few years. There can be no question that the brain, being nourished by the blood stream, should benefit when that stream carries the vital, living elements brought about by eating organically produced food. I can notice it quite definitely. This is not boasting, because it is due not to myself, but to a completely outside factor, my food. You can do the same thing.

We have received hundreds of letters from readers of *Organic Gardening* testifying to the remarkable results they have obtained by applying the organic method in their gardens. They have better plants and less plant pests. I can remember only a few letters telling of improvement in personal health. One a few days ago from Mrs. H. J. Schauer of Roseville, California, said, "and since we have learned to raise our fruit and vegetables the organic way our health has improved one hundred per cent."

There were a half dozen letters from persons who had secured benefits from eating sunflower seeds. Of course, *Organic Gardening* has been published less than three years, so that our readers have not practiced this method as long as we have. We *do* expect, from now on, to hear of many cases of such health benefits resulting from eating organically produced food.

If medical science could investigate this subject I believe they would find that organically produced food stimulates and adds to our intestinal flora. This flora consists of bacteria, living organisms, which take an extremely important part in digesting our food. Recently at the University of Wisconsin experiments showed that some vitamins are actually manufactured in the intestines by bacteria. This digestive process is aided by enzymes, which are living substances, but not bacteria. In other words the act of digestion is a biologic process, not a chemical one. Food produced organically is more alive and contains more living elements, which gradually build up an intestinal flora with tremendous power of digestibility.

It is the same with soil. What is the measure of fertility of earth? Its microbial population. A soil extremely fertile and profuse with bacteria and fungi will digest a gunny sack in a few months. A chemicalized soil, with one-half the amount of soil microbes, will take years to do the same thing. Aristotle called earthworms the intestines of the soil. He was right, but he did not know about bacteria. The microscope wasn't invented yet. Together, the earthworm and the microbe represent the earth's stomach. They digest the food for plants. I wouldn't be surprised if they work in a team, supplementing each other's activities. For example, bacteria do not like an acid condition. The earthworm with its calciferous glands is a powerful factor in keeping the soil properly sweetened.

If all the statesmen of the world and all the government officials could eat food produced organically from fertile soil rich in minerals, the possibility of future wars would be greatly diminished.

[31]

8. Teeth and the Organic Method

The following is an article from the February, 1952, issue of *Prevention*:

One of the first dividends our family received from the practicing of the organic method and the eating of foods raised organically was a noticeable improvement in our teeth. There were less and less cavities every time we went to the dentist. In the case of our youngest child, Nina, who is now thirteen, the condition of her teeth is perfect. She does not have a single cavity in any of her teeth. This was made possible in her case because she was only about three years old when we began to eat food raised organically. In my own case I have not had a cavity in five years. Hundreds of our readers have also noted a wonderful improvement in their teeth. Typical is the case of a family of three that came to see me recently, who told that where they used to have a yearly dental bill of about a hundred dollars, it is now reduced to about ten dollars, and consists only of routine cleaning. Only a few days ago a woman from Rhode Island told me that she stopped having cavities five years ago, after she began eating organically grown food. And the peculiar thing is, far from their entire diet is organically produced. Usually the organic portion consists only of the vegetables that they raise in their own garden.

Some purchase organically produced food through the mails. It is amazing what a small amount of organically produced food will do for the health of a person.

Permit me to quote an item from the *Field Magazine,* published in England, dated January 6, 1945:

"I was interested in your letter from *Dental Surgeon,* because my seven-year-old son and I have only just paid a routine visit to the dentist. He seemed quite unusually impressed by the excellence of my son's teeth and asked me if he had had any special diet. I told him: No, that he had eaten no meat (including eggs) up to the age of three years, but since then had eaten meat and exactly what he liked. I added, however, that we grew as much of our food as possible on composted soil and that for more than his lifetime we have never used an ounce of artificial fertilizers.

" 'You have given me the answer,' said the dentist. 'Now I understand why he has teeth like that.'

"In my own case, my teeth used to collect huge quantities of tartar. Every year it had to be scraped off. We began using compost instead of artificials toward the end of 1936. When I went to my dentist in 1942, after a lapse (I am ashamed to say) of two-and-a-half years, I expected a terrific scraping to occur. There was no tartar to remove. Another two years elapsed before I went again, this last time. There was a very little tartar behind two teeth, and that was all.

"We have used compost for just about eight years, and for the last five of those years my teeth have lost their unpleasant habit of collecting tartar. Is this a coincidence? It might be. But I was telling this story to someone else, and she has had exactly the same experience. Incidentally, I asked the dentist if wartime diet could have anything to do with it. He did not think it had, because he finds now just as much tartar collecting on his other patients' teeth as before the war."

(L. F. Easterbrook)

Note: Bone meal plus organically grown food would be a 99 per cent deterrent to the getting of dental cavities.

9. Our Barn Rats

I MUST REPORT to you a piece of evidence, something that happened which showed how healthful the regular consumption of an organically grown diet could be. Let me tell you the story of our barn rats!

When we bought our farm about 25 years ago, we inherited the mangiest lot of barn rats that ever infested a barn. And I could see the reason for it. They had available to them as food a pretty low order of grain—grain grown in an exhausted piece of infertile clay soil—dead end as far as soils are concerned—a pretty raw deal it was, if you should ask me, even for rats.

And the farmer tenant's cows would never take any prizes at the country fair. They were knobby, misshapen and scrubby. The chickens were dying by the dozen, and not of old age. The farmer didn't have enough energy to give them a decent burial, for you could see them lying dead under the corncrib where he threw them. There is an old saying—poor land, poor cattle, poor people. To which I would add, poor rats.

My introduction to these rats came one evening shortly after we moved onto the farm, when I went into the barn on a tour of inspection. I threw on the lights and the sudden blinding glare surprised a few of the rodents which were eating at a long trough of fodder intended for the steers. These rats struck me as being terribly starved and emaciated. They were painfully skinny, their bones showing through their mangy skins like those of a glue-factory horse. I wasn't experienced with rats in those days, but any untaught neophyte in the art of observing run-of-the-mill rodents could have seen that these were the worst specimens of their kind you could find anywhere. They looked terribly dissatisfied—probably over the fact that the farmer had not been feeding them the way he should have. If they could have gotten their diseased teeth into his pants, they would have written a message there he would never forget.

I threw a stick and they began to run—a nervous, frantic, snarling sort of run. It didn't take a genius to see that they were savagely confused in their outlook, that there was a rebellious spirit apparent in their general attitude, that they were a mean, murderous lot of rats.

Well, sir, if you are a sir, and madame, if you hate rats and rat stories, for which I humbly apologize, the curtain descends and remains down for three years. Now it is Act II, as we say in the theatre. During those three years we practiced the organic method assiduously. We fertilized our soil with compost. We raised its organic matter and humus content appreciably. We treated the good earth with reverence and kindness. We did not apply poisonous insecticides of any kind. We used no chemical fertilizers. The land became healed. No more chickens died. In these three years the regeneration of the soil showed itself in our wonderfully healthy crops.

Now the curtain goes up again, and we are in Act III. What was my surprise one night, when I put the lights on in the barn, to see some sleek-looking, well-nourished, contented, thoroughly stabilized rats, dining at the selfsame troughs in the same steer section of the same barn. The last time, as you will recall, those rats were eating, but this time they were dining. One of them gently turned toward me and blinked its eyes as if to say, "Hello there, stranger, where have *you* been all this time, and what brings you here this time o' night? What can I *do* for you?"

"What can I do for you?" I countered, as I took a stick, aimed it carefully, and threw it at him with the strength of a man who does not get headaches. You may not believe my eyes, but it's the God's honest truth. I can still see that rat vividly today, because he had such a whimsical, George Gobel quality about him. He looked at me with a pudgy, squinty-eyed sort of expression, as if he was greatly amused by what I had done, while he slowly but surely dodged the missile that was coming toward him. His relaxed mind was able to coordinate his actions to a split-second response, because he moved just enough to miss the piece of wood by a thirty-second of an inch.

"Now, why did you do that?" he seemed to ask, as he waddled away. I'm sure he chuckled. I could hear it as plain as the scratching of my pen right this minute.

Now this is not a fish story, and I am not sitting on a hot radiator as I write. (That tends to draw the blood away from the brain.) I'm in the full possession of all my God-given faculties, and every word I have said is the Gospel truth, as are all my adventures related in this book. By this time the rest of the rats began to move slowly away, evidently extremely fascinated by the amusing pantomime they had just witnessed.

[36]

At the time, I didn't realize the significance of the little drama I had witnessed, but as I lay in bed that night, it hit me with the impact of a sledge-hammer blow, or that of a bale of organically grown hay weighing a couple of hundred pounds, whichever carries the most impact.

In my original writing of this I used only a sledge hammer, but I began to figure that this is such a common cliché that I ought to do something about it. It so happens, however, that I am a cliché lover, so I kept the sledge hammer and added the bale of hay for originality. Where was I? Oh, yes!

Those rats were being fed an organically grown diet without the harmful effects of chemical fertilizers. No matter how careful one is on a farm, the rats are sure to get at the crops somehow. In handling sacks of grain one always spills some of it on the floor of the barn, and there is always an open sack beckoning to a more-than-willing rat. And if the sack isn't open the rats play a game called "Open up the Sack," which will accomplish the same thing.

Slowly over those three years my rats and their progeny were getting all the benefits of an organically produced diet.

Come to think of it, the rats that I had the honor of meeting in that third year were perhaps of the tenth generation: organically fed, that is. They were endowed with a grand aristocratic heritage, and if I make my rats sound royal, it is being done intentionally, for they are healthier than any king or queen living that I know of. Their great-great-great grandparents, back to God-knows-what degree of great-great-great-great-ness, had had the benefit of this highly mineralized and vitaminized organic diet. I am unashamedly proud of my rats, and will stack them against those of any other farmer for a hundred miles around, or even farther: I would also like to say to farmers who have rats living with them, either feed them properly, or destroy them. No in-between measures are Christian.

All this happened between about 1941 and 1944. In 1949 we had the opportunity to witness a scientific proof of what a healthful diet could do to the health of rats. As president of the Soil and Health Foundation I was associated with Dr. Ehrenfried Pfeiffer in an experiment in the feeding of mice at his laboratory at Threefold Farms, Spring Valley, N. Y., the results of which were reported in Bulletin 2 of the Soil and Health Foundation, dated November 1, 1949. The experiment was undertaken in order to find out whether the treatment of soil with organic materials or with chemical fertilizers would show a difference in the feeding and health values of products grown under such farming methods, and various groups of mice were fed by food raised by these different methods.

It was found that the death rate from fighting was distinctly higher in the chemical fertilizer group than in the organic one. There were more irritable and nervous mice in the chemical fertilizer group. I saw this for myself when I visited this experiment. The mice are kept six in a box and each box is divided into two rooms, because a mouse likes to sleep in one room and eat in another. In the partition between the two sections is a tiny door which is wide enough to permit one mouse at a time to walk through with comfort. When we opened up the chemically fertilized mouse box, that is, took off the top cover and let the light in, the mice became so frantic that they started to run. Two or three of them tried to go through the door at the same time, getting stuck and remaining there squealing and howling. But when we opened up the boxes in which the organically fed mice were kept, this did not happen. The mice continued nonchalantly about their business. It was interesting that the same thing happened time and again as we opened up the boxes. The chemically fed mice were invariably nervous while the organically fed ones were invariably relaxed.

Of the causes of death, stomach disorders were prevalent in the chemically fertilized group to an extent of about 16 per cent, but only about 3 per cent in the organic group. The results of this experiment showed that the survival rate of the organic group was markedly higher than that of the chemical fertilizer group: 32.63 per cent as against 21.38 per cent in the first generation. In another strain of mice the survival rate was 64.41 per cent in the organic group as against 35.39 per cent in the chemical group. Larger litters were born to the organically fed mice.

Some time later an interesting experiment was performed. It is a known fact that certain chemicals when rubbed on the skin produce cancer. One of these chemicals was applied to the skin of all the mice. On that of the chemically fertilized fed group, cancer of the skin reached as high as 71 per cent, but in the organically fed group only 45 per cent contracted it.

Another proof of what I observed in my barn was demonstrated by Sir Robert McCarrison at Coonoor, in India in 1927. He was Director of Nutrition Research for all of India.

He decided to find out if rats could be endowed with health equal to that enjoyed by the Hunzas through feeding the rodents on a similar diet. One group was, consequently, fed the diet upon which the Hunzukuts and other healthy peoples of Northern India, such as the Sikhs, Pathans and Mahrattas, subsist. Another group of rats was fed the poor diet of the Southern

India rice-eaters, the Bengali and Madrassi. In his aforementioned book, McCarrison referred to a nutritional authority, McCay, who twenty-five years before had written, "As we pass from the Northwest region of the Punjab down the Gangetic Plain to the coast of Bengal, there is a gradual fall in the stature, body weight, stamina and efficiency of the people. In accordance with this decline in many characteristics it is of the utmost significance that there is an accompanying gradual fall in the nutritive value of the dietaries." And so McCarrison found it.

A third group of rats was subjected to the diet of the lower classes of England, containing white bread, margarine, sweetened tea, a little boiled milk, cabbage and potatoes, tinned meats and jam. The results were startling. McCarrison described the first group as being *hunzarized*. "During the past two and a quarter years," he stated, "there has been no case of illness in this 'universe' of albino rats, no death from natural causes in the adult stock, and but for a few accidental deaths, no infantile mortality. Both clinically and at post-mortem examination this stock has been shown to be remarkably free from disease. But the Bengali group of rats suffered from a wide variety of diseases which involved every organ of the body such as the nose, eyes, ears, stomach, lungs, bladder, kidneys, intestines, the blood, glands, nerves and reproductive organs. In addition, they suffered from loss of hair, malformed and crooked spines, poor teeth, ulcers, boils and became vicious and irritable."

The "English" rats also developed most of these troubles. They were nervous and apt to bite their attendants; they lived unhappily together and by the sixtieth day of the experiment they began to kill and eat the weaker ones amongst them.

[40]

Before I leave this chapter I would like to compare my own care with that of the two phases of my barn rats.

Phase One

About 25 years ago I was not health-conscious. I was eating a typical modern diet, with lots of bread, cakes and other starches with an over-consumption of sweets, and with no taking of vitamins or minerals. My weight was about 205. Today I am 168. I did not do any walking then. Today I walk at least an hour a day. At that time I was very nervous, and used to explode with anger at employees who made mistakes.

I really was a nervous wreck, like one of my old barn rats, and only 39 years old. I recall one time going to a movie with my wife, and in the picture there was loud noises of airplanes. I couldn't stand it—I had to rush out of the theatre.

Phase Two

Today at 71 I have become wonderfully stabilized and can stand any kind of noise, retaining a serene poise in emergencies. I practically never get angry regardless of the provocation. A few years ago I engaged in a debate on fluoridation with a dentist at a P.T.A. meeting. There was a large crowd. I took the side against fluoridation. In the course of the proceedings the dentist, a poorly nourished man, I am sure, called me a liar. I sat there smiling, twiddling my thumbs. Excitement ran around the room. A newspaper reporter came over and expressed his admiration at my calmness. Instead of getting angry, I answered that dentist with facts against fluoridation.

The next morning one of the school directors phoned me and wanted to know if I desired a public apology.

[41]

But I said no. I am not vindictive. I am a happy, tolerant man, and for it I give a great deal of credit to my diet.

10. Wheat and the Birds

Here is something I wrote in *Prevention,* March, 1952:

On our farm we raised wheat for the last two years in an experiment in large cylinders, some of which were fertilized with chemical fertilizers and some by our organic method, using only organic matter, plus mild ground-up phosphate and potash rock. What was our surprise one day that the wheat was heading out to ripeness when a flock of birds came to eat the heads, but they went only to the plots containing the wheat raised organically. They would not touch those that were grown with chemical fertilizers. Evidently an animal's taste is more selective than a human being's, and the birds could easily see that the organically produced wheat seed was much tastier, a sign that it contained more vitamins, minerals and general nourishment.

11. Sunflower Seeds

IN THE latter part of 1941 an amazing situation in Deaf Smith County, Texas, was brought to the attention of the American public. It was discovered that the inhabitants of that county, living mainly in and around Hereford, had remarkably healthy teeth with the almost complete absence of dental caries. Authorities who investigated found that the Deaf Smith Countians had teeth superior to anything known anywhere in the world. You might say that tooth decay there was practically non-existent. Even the horses, dogs and cats in that region of Texas had perfect teeth. When strangers moved into this section their dental troubles vanished. New cavities did not form. The old ones glazed over and progressed no further.

A study of the locality revealed the fact that underlying the soil was a rich deposit of lime (calcium) and phosphorus with a trace of fluorine. Since all soils have been formed from their underlying rock structure in a weathering process extending over eons of time, it was found that the soil in and around Hereford was rich in lime and phosphorus and contained some fluorine. These three elements are extremely important in connection with the formation of tooth and bone, and since the food raised in Deaf Smith County soil absorbs sizable amounts of these substances, it gives the residents of this county healthy tooth and bone structure. Farmers of this section bring in spindly cows and steers from across the border in Mexico and after pasturing and feeding them with local produce build them up into fine big-boned animals.

A New England dentist avidly read the reports about the teeth in this celebrated county and his imagination ran completely away from the daily grind of drills, forceps and bicuspids. He cleverly reasoned that if he could find some food that was plentiful and which contained those three elements, namely calcium, phosphorus and fluorine in sufficient quantities, he might be

[43]

able to accomplish the same purpose without causing a gold-rush on Deaf Smith County. That man is Dr. S. G. Harootian, connected with the Worcester State Hospital, in Mass.

He found such a food—the bones of beef cattle ground fine as flour. In an astounding nine-month experiment with nine mental patients at his hospital he absolutely arrested the formation of cavities. Only one new cavity was formed in all that time. These patients were chosen because of their notoriously poor dental history. They were fed a capsule consisting of five grains of bone flour three times daily, along with their regular diet.

In the case of one of the patients, a filling was removed so as to expose the cavity to the ravages of the elements. It was continually packed with food debris, naturally. This would have been suicide for that particular tooth under ordinary conditions, but this wasn't an ordinary condition. Under the bone flour regimen that tooth did not decay. This experiment received a great deal of publicity and was written up in many journals. One of the large meat packers advises that they are conducting tests with bone flour to see if it has any adverse effects on the human body. It is already on sale in some places.

The dental profession feels that it is mostly the fluorine that is the agent which keeps down tooth decay. In 1944 the N. Y. Institute of Clinical Pathologists started a most important experiment. The drinking water of Newburgh, N. Y. is having sodium fluorine added to it in extremely tiny quantities, as too much would be toxic to human beings. The neighboring city of Kingston will act as the control by not having anything added to its water. This will go on for ten years. In the meantime the teeth of all children between five and twelve years old in these towns will be examined each year, as well as those over 50. The fluorinated water will no doubt have some beneficial effect on the people of Newburgh, but I don't think this experiment goes far enough. Half the people in this town should also be given foods rich in calcium and phosphorus, so that the full effect of the findings in Deaf Smith County may be tested.

Many tribes of American Indians realized that bones made a valuable adjunct to the diet. They favored the bones of fish which they ground into a flour and mixed with various foods.

As a spectator I was irresistibly fascinated by these momentous happenings. For several years on our farm we had been growing sunflowers and feeding the seeds of this plant to our chickens. Poultry authorities speak highly of this seed as a conditioner of barnyard fowl. Parrots live on them almost exclusively and seem to lead a contented existence. We had never thought of eating these seeds ourselves but when I heard about Deaf Smith County and Dr. Harootian's ingenious experiment the thought occurred to me to check up the food-value analysis of sunflower seeds. To my amazement the ash of the seed showed a tremendous quantity of phosphorus (35 per cent), calcium (seven and one-half per cent) and a trace of fluorine.

I started to eat the seeds, a couple of heaping handfuls every day, but did not adjust anything else in my diet. My dentist had found only one tiny tooth cavity in about three years so I wasn't thinking in terms of dental improvement. But about four days later I noticed something that was truly startling. My gums had stopped bleeding. They say that four out of five suffer from pink tooth brush, (actually the figures are more nearly one out of five). If this condition is not checked it may eventually lead to something far more serious than mere tooth cavities, namely, the dreaded *pyorrhea* and the loss of all teeth. When I used to eat an apple I could sometimes see a slight bloody imprint on the white pulp. This embarrassing condition cleared up nicely so I stuck faithfully to my sunflower seeds.

About a week later a slight intermittent quiver in my left eye went away. I usually suffered from this only in the winter when there was little opportunity for exercise or sunshine. As this is written two winters later I am glad to report that it has not returned, thanks to the fact that I still eat sunflower seeds practically every day.

My eyes are not my strongest point. In the winter I would have trouble in walking on snow-blanketed roads. Before I became aware of the value of eating sunflower seeds I left the house on the farm one day for a walk but had to return after being out only a moment, as the excessive brightness of the snow interfered with my vision. In fact, it made the snow seem a pink color. After being on the sunflower diet for about a month I noticed I could walk in the snow without distress. A little while later my car broke down and I had to walk over a mile on a snowed-up highway in bright sunshine with no trouble at all for the first three-quarters of the way. On the last stretch the eyes smarted a little.

The sunflower seed is loaded down with vitamin B. The oil found in sunflower seeds is very rich in vitamin A which is known to be essential to robust eye health. I noticed also that my skin seemed to be getting smoother. This doesn't seem to be unreasonable because calcium and vitamin A are specifics for a good strong epidermis. Dr. Bogert in her book "Nutrition and Physical Fitness" says, "Hard, dry skin, which may be inflamed or show a peculiar eruption, has been noted

[46]

in poor people of China, Ceylon and East Africa on diets low in vitamin A, and the skin returned to normal when cod-liver oil was given. Skin lesions in infantile eczema are also said to clear up after giving amounts of vitamin A." If the eating of sunflower seeds will give Milady a smooth skin, there is a great future for them.

Recently Drs. H. C. Sherman and H. L. Campbell, of Columbia University, reported to the National Academy of Sciences that the proper amount of vitamin A intake is extremely important to the well-being of the individual. In fact these doctors declare that it postpones aging and actually increases the length of life of the individual.

I now decided to see if the eating of sunflower seeds would have the same effect on the bleeding gums of others. I therefore furnished these seeds to four girls employed in the shops of an electric manufacturing company of which I am vice-president. Within ten days two of them reported complete success; no more blood on toothbrushes. One girl claimed 50 per cent improvement. This girl stated her tongue did not seem to be coated anymore. The fourth girl estimated a 75 per cent improvement. I have checked with three of these girls a year later and the improvements are holding.

I have gone over many books on nutrition and nowhere have I seen reference made to the value of the sunflower seed in the diet. In lists giving the vitamin content of foods, the sunflower is usually left out. Evidently this is because it has always been a bird and chicken food. Thus it seems to be left completely out of the calculations of the best nutritionists. It is the forgotten food, if there ever was one.

In a bulletin on sunflower seeds written by the late well-known nutritionist Harvey W. Wiley (U.S. Dept. of Agriculture Bulletin No. 60, published in 1901) he

says that there was an old idea that the eating of sunflower seeds would cure rheumatism. However, Mr.
Wiley stated further that there was no evidence that it
would. Many of the so-called home remedies have
proven unusually effective when checked by the medical profession. Digitalis for heart-disease, for example,
is a drug obtained from the fox-glove flower. A physician discovered an old woman using it and on checking
found it remarkably successful in his work. It is now a
standard medical remedy. There are dozens of other
similar cases. In fact there is an entire field of botanical
drugs used by many physicians. So perhaps, even as a
specific for rheumatism, the sunflower cannot be waved
away without some experimental testing. Our folklore is
rich in cases of wholesome, simple cures by means of
various plants.

There are many reasons why the sunflower seed is
a valuable food and should be included in everyone's
daily diet. In the first place nature protects it with a
casing. It therefore stores well and loses very little vitamin value for long periods. When you remove the outer
shell you have a concentrated bit of healthy nourishment. It tastes almost as delicious a year after harvesting as on the day it was cut down. I have eaten with
relish raw wheat seed on harvest day, but a month later
it has already lost some of its palatability.

Secondly, you eat the sunflower seed raw. Nutritionists all agree that cooking, however skillfully done,
destroys some of the vitamins. It is not factoryized or
processed food. It comes to you in virgin form.

This plant is one of the easiest to grow. You have
never heard of anyone spraying poisons on it because
it is very hardy and is highly resistant to disease.

Now we come to a very remarkable fact about the
sunflower. As soon as the head is formed it always faces

[48]

the sun. This is a phenomenon called *heliotropism*. In the morning the head faces the east. As the sun swings in its orbit across the heavens, the sunflower head turns with it gradually, until, late in the afternoon, it is facing due west to absorb the few last rays of the dying sun. Sometimes before the sun comes up next morning the head turns completely back to start the process all over again. Every farmer boy knows this. In other words it is just drenched with sun-vitality. Perhaps that is the reason it wards off the diseases which plague other plants. Another possible reason for the potency of this little seed is that from such a small speck, there comes in a few weeks time quite a quantity of green material, much greater than that of any other of our food crop plants in proportion to size of seed. Nature, therefore, must pack this tiny kernel full of powerful stuff.

Due to the fact that the plants are so attentive to the sun, the seeds are very rich in vitamin D, which is known as the sun vitamin. Yet you can search high and low in authoritative lists of vitamins and you will not find the sunflower listed. It became lost in the shuffle somewhere and requires a new deal. Under vitamin D, you will usually find cod-liver oil, canned salmon, egg yolk, liver, cheese, cream and milk, but no sunflower seed.

In the U. S. it is sometimes grown as a border to beautify a garden and the seeds are later thrown away. A friend of mine admitted to this crime. He didn't know whether you eat the seed shelled or with the jackets. I have since discovered many other persons who were guilty of the same uncertainty. You throw away the shell, of course.

The American Indian found copious use for the seed of the sunflower which he employed as food, hair oil and soap. Members of the Lewis and Clark expedition found much evidence of this. In their journal for July 17, 1805, when they were in Montana there is recorded the following:

"Along the bottoms, which have a covering of high grass, we observe the *sunflower* blooming in great abundance. The Indians of the Missouri, more especially those who do not cultivate maize, make great use of the seed of this plant for bread, or in thickening their soup. They first patch and then pound it between two stones, until it is reduced to a fine meal. Sometimes they add a portion of water, and drink it thus diluted; at other times they add a sufficient proportion of marrow-grease to reduce it to the consistency of common dough, and eat it in that manner. This last composition we preferred to all the rest, and thought it at that time a very palatable dish."

Note the use of marrow-grease, a product made from bones. Columbus also noted how popular the sunflower was with the Indians and was instrumental in introducing it into Europe. Today, while this seed is so popular in many parts of Europe, it is practically unknown in this country as a food for human beings.

In 1955, there developed in my left eye a slight quiver, which did not seem to want to go away. That was bad for an editor of a health magazine. I let a few weeks pass, thinking that, like a ship that passes in the night, it would go away. I closed my eyes to it, but it persisted.

I thought back to my pamphlet *Sunflower Seed—The Miracle Food,* written about ten years ago, and re-read the following in it: "About a week later (that is, after beginning to eat sunflower seeds) a slight intermittent quiver in my left eye went away. I usually suffered from this only in the winter, when there was little opportunity for exercise or sunshine. As this is

[50]

written two winters later I am glad to report that it has not returned, thanks to the fact that I still eat sunflower seeds practically every day."

Well, I seemed to have gotten careless, and had stopped eating sunflower seeds somewhere along the line. So I began eating them again. But I had none of our own organically-raised ones. The previous year's crop of them had been fed to the chickens. So I began to eat some hulled seeds that we had around the house and that had been purchased some months before. I ate them for several weeks, but nothing happened.

Along about October our new crop ripened and I began to eat our own seeds. Within three days my eye quiver vanished, but before I could start crowing, that is about two days after that, it returned in fairly full vigor.

"Hm," said I. "This is more serious than I thought. But I must track this thing down. There must be *some* cause." There always are causes and they can be found if one keeps one's mind at it. It is a matter of a little thinking plus a little of trial and error.

The next thing that I tried to incriminate was my pillow. Years ago I had a pain in the neck which evidently was caused solely by sleeping on a pillow. Crooking the head causes a bend in the jugular vein of the neck. The veins become wrinkled at the point of bend, and congestion of the blood circulation occurs there. There is not a free flow of blood to and from the head. Within a few days of learning to sleep flat, the pain completely cleared up—but completely. A few months ago I heard one of the girls in our circulation department complaining of a pain in the neck. I described my own experience to her and in a very short time she completely rid herself of it—solely by sleeping without a pillow.

[51]

Here again I had gotten careless, and a few years ago had resorted to the pillow again. Nothing happened by sleeping on a pillow this time; that is, the pain in the neck did not return. But now I began to suspect the pillow in connection with my eye quiver. If there was a congestion in the mechanism that feeds blood to the head, perhaps the eyes weren't getting enough blood. So I began to sleep without a pillow. A few weeks went by but the quiver remained—and I was exactly where I started.

I noticed, however, that when I took my glasses off, the quiver was less marked. I don't want to give you a wrong impression. The eye did not quiver constantly—it was an intermittent thing. But with the glasses off it was a little more intermittent. My glasses could have something to do with it, thought I. The next day saw me at the optometrist, my personal friend. "It could be one of two things," he said. "Either it is a calcium deficiency, or your left eye has either improved or gotten worse, that is, the lens for your left eye might need correction."

Now let's go back to sunflower seeds. Although they did not cure my eye quiver, I observed a remarkable effect through eating them. About five years ago, a heavy book fell on my left foot, hitting the right half of the big toe-nail, and blacking that part of it. After about six months, as the blackness did not show any signs of going away, I went to an Allentown surgeon who treated it by cutting the right half of the nail right down to the base. I would come to see him each week, and as the nail grew back, he would continue to cut it back. But the blackness remained. After a few months of this unsuccessful treatment, I stopped going.

For four years I watched that nail and the right half of it continued to remain black. There was abso-

[52]

lutely no pain to it, and I felt a feeling of security due to my excellent nutrition. I knew that my vitamin E was keeping the circulation active in my feet. One day, early in the morning, while I was indulging in my usual one-hour walk on the soft turf of the Allentown Fair Grounds, whom should I meet but my old surgeon friend, riding his horse! He stopped, and we exchanged a few words. I told him that my nail was still black and asked him if there was any danger in it. He said absolutely not. I was resigned to carry a black toe nail to the grave.

But then I began to eat sunflower seeds in an attempt to stop my eye quiver. Within about ten days I noticed a lighter region in the newly grown nail, only about a sixteenth of an inch from its base. I kept watching it. Gradually the lighter section kept going higher and higher until, about a week ago, it reached to the top. The blackness is completely gone and the color is only slightly darker than that of a natural nail. What do you think of that? I can attribute it to nothing else than the effect of eating sunflower seeds, my own organically-grown ones. There must be something extremely potent about them. They are a seed from which a huge amount of plant tissue will grow. They contain a living element, a germ, which represents life and which you do not get when you eat such foods as lettuce or carrots. In the old Czarist days, Russian soldiers were given what was called an iron ration—sunflower seeds. I do not know whether this custom has carried over into modern times.

I like another thing about the sunflower seed. The sunflower plant usually turns with the sun as it grows, the head containing the seeds always being exposed to it. It thus becomes sun-drenched. A friend has an electric machine that tests the electric potential of plants.

[53]

He has found that foods growing in the sun contain a higher electric potential than foods like the potato that grow in the ground. He also has found that apples growing on the outside of the tree, that get the sun, have much more electric potential than those growing in the interior of the tree where it is shady.

The ash of the sunflower seed shows a tremendous amount of phosphorus (35%), calcium (7½%) and a trace of fluorine. The sunflower seed has more vitamin B than wheat seed and it is very rich in vitamin A.

In my opinion the sunflower seed, unroasted and unsalted, is dynamite in its wonderful effect on the body. It is a specific for the eyes.

I will eat a handful of sunflower seeds every day for the rest of my life, and advise you to do likewise—about 50 or 60 of them a day should be enough. And if you have the tiniest bit of grass you ought to grow your own sunflower plants organically. The sunflower plant is the easiest thing to grow. If you don't have any compost, use a liberal amount of dried blood and bone meal, which are available at chain stores, nurseries and seed stores.

A word of caution. The bone meal that you buy for use as a fertilizer is not for human consumption. It may contain disease organisms that are harmful to a weakened human body. Another word of caution— some people have trouble cracking sunflower seeds with their teeth, either through having false teeth or because it might result in chipping sensitive teeth or separating the two front teeth. I would suggest two things: Either soak the seeds in cold water with their shells on, or open them with a pair of pliers. Will someone develop a little hand tool that could open these seeds easily?

In conclusion, I have related three things in one package. The cure of the quiver, the improvement of

[54]

my eyesight, and the getting rid of the black toe-nail. If I continue improving at this rate I will live a long time. It is my ambition to live to be 102 years and one day. Why the extra day? I was born in 1898. If I live to be 102 years and one day, I will have lived in three centuries.

12. The Rodale Diet

In the April, 1952, *Prevention* I began to explore the subject of pesticide residues on fruits and vegetables, and began a method of preferring foods that were more or less protected from these poisonous sprays. Pineapple is an example because of its heavy skin protection. Coconuts are another fruit that is similarly protected, and cantaloupe. Peas would be part of this diet because the spray goes on the pod, and corn is more or less protected by its sheath. So are nuts and sunflower seeds.

13. A Low-Poison Diet

I would like to discuss a plan by which you can severely limit the amount of chemical additives in your food. If you will adopt my idea of eating no foods made in a factory, with a few safe exceptions, such as packaged raisins, you will already have eliminated a tremendous percentage of additive chemicals you have been consuming up to now. You will have stopped eating cheeses and other dairy products. Cheeses not only contain emulsifiers and other chemicals, but they are also heavily loaded with salt. Do not drink milk—this is made in a factory, for what is a cow if not a factory, the way they have overbred her? Besides milk contains residues of DDT and penicillin, often hydrogen peroxide as a bacteria killer, oat gum as an antioxidant, and sometimes other chemicals.

The remaining categories of foods that are chemically tainted are the fruits and vegetables that have been sprayed with poisonous insecticides. Don't think that if you cut off the skins, you are avoiding these poisons, because they are usually absorbed into the interior of the fruit. The problem here is to see how much we can eliminate in these two categories to cut our insecticide consumption to a low level.

Pears receive far less insecticide than apples. Therefore, cut out apples entirely and eat pears only occasionally, or not at all. If you buy in health food stores you can get raisins, figs and dates that are pretty safe.

Nuts: This is rather a large group, and a very healthy one. Their hard shells protect them from poison sprays of all kinds. The list includes walnut, brazil nut, hazel nut, filbert, Indian or Pinyon nuts, peanuts and chestnuts. The peanut grows underground and therefore is doubly protected. I knew a man who lived to be over 90 and in his last 30 years lived almost exclusively on nuts.

Do not buy shelled nuts. They are cheaper and healthier if purchased in their shells. In the factories chemicals are sometimes used to shell nuts.

Coconut: Another food protected by a heavy shell is the coconut, which is rich in minerals. In many warm countries it forms the main staple of the diet.

Pineapple: Do not buy the canned variety. Its heavy

skin protects this fruit from poisonous insecticides that seep through the thin skins of other fruits. The pineapple is very rich in vitamin C, protein and enzymes which aid the digestion.

Bananas: Bananas have a rather protective skin, but I would say regarding bananas, moderation—only about 2 or 3 a week.

Watermelon, Honeydew, Cantaloupe: All are protected by heavy skins and are excellent foods. We scoop some of the inside pulp of the cantaloupe along with the seeds and break them up in a blender, as a very satisfying and nutritious drink. The seeds are a potent item of nutrition.

Avocado: It has a thick dark green skin, with a meaty melon-like pulp, and is known to be a very healthy food.

Pumpkin and Squash: Can be served mashed like turnips or potatoes, or can be cubed and boiled. Europeans go in for pumpkin soup. Pumpkin can be mixed into a blender to make drinks of various kinds.

Potatoes: Both white and sweet potatoes grow underground where they do not receive direct applications of insecticides. I highly recommend sweet potatoes. Potatoes are not half as fattening as bread and cake.

Beets and Carrots: Both grow underground and are a desirable addition to your diet.

Eggplant: Its thick skin repels many dangerous chemicals. It is rich in vitamins A and C.

Peas and Beans: There are 5 or 6 items in this category, all protected by their pods.

Radishes, Turnips, Parsnips: All grow underground.

Wild Rice, Brown Rice, Corn: Corn is well protected by its sheath. Wild rice grows under natural conditions and brown rice has had a minimum of chemical contacts.

Sunflower and Pumpkin Seeds: These two seeds happen to be most marvelous food, well protected from chemicals. For anyone aiming at developing the highest degree of health, these seeds are strongly recommended. The seed is a live food. When planted in the soil an enormous amount of plant tissue will grow out of it. It therefore contains rare mineral, vitamin and life-giving substances that are highly desirable for optimum nutrition. Seeds can be obtained, shelled or hulled for easy eating, in all health food stores.

Olive and Other Oils: Olive oil, a tablespoonful at each meal, will keep a stomach ulcer under control and is a worthwhile item of diet for general health. The olive tree lives for thousands of years. There may be something in the sap that promotes health and longevity. The Italians thrive on it.

There are more foods that are protected from the spray guns, but these are all I can think of right now. Of course, you will not want to stick 100 per cent with these foods. But with regard to others, moderation is the word. You will in time feel the benefits of a diet very low in chemical additives.

You will of course add to the above fresh meats, fish, and eggs.

14. Avoid Wheat Products

I AM DEFINITELY against any wheat or rye product for human consumption, and am never afraid to express my attitude, which, as a rule, brings down a shower of verbal brick-bats and dressingdowns from the whole-wheat school of health, and especially from those who make their own bread from organically raised wheat. To them it has become a sacred ritual—a symbol. To me it is a matter of searching for the truth. What is the best program for a person who wishes to live to 120? I say, don't eat bread. It is the worst form of starch. I put bananas at the head of the starch list, and somewhat further down . . . potatoes, but bread? I wouldn't even give it any place in the list. It is not edible starch. It is for paste. I eat the wheat germ and perhaps the bran portion . . . but not the paste portion of the wheat.

15. Bread Positively Cited Common Cause of Colds

What is wrong with wheat? First of all it is one of the most fattening foods. The *Esquire* reducing diet which consists of merely cutting out wheat and rye guarantees a loss of about 20 pounds in two months. Bread is one of the most common causes of colds, a fact proven by medical researches which we have cited time and time again. If you suffer from a stuffed-up nose or head, cut out bread and see what an improvement will come about at once. Bread fills people up, it gives them a false feeling of hunger satisfaction. Thus they eat less of fruit, vegetables and other important foods. Bread is difficult of digestion by the human stomach. Dr. Alvarez of the Mayo Clinic showed that bread can pass through the whole of the small intestine without becoming digested at all. Bread requires a large production of digestive juices for its complete solution. The protein of the bread especially is defectively absorbed by the intestine. A significant medically proven fact is that whole wheat bread interferes with the absorption of other foods. I have found this to be so in my case.

Bread is fine for cows who have 4 stomachs and keep chewing their cud. But in the human digestive system, because it is not completely digested, it ferments or rots.

It is one of the most common causes of constipation. Wheat causes rickets in children where there is an overconsumption of this type of food. It is the underlying factor in a disease of children called celiac disease, which is increasing alarmingly. The abdomen becomes distended, there is fat in the stools. The doctor orders an immediate elimination of all wheat products. Wheat has been found to be one of the causes of tooth cavities. Wheat products are one of the common causes of asthma.

16. Bread Held Responsible for Several Diseases

One physician discovered that bread was one of the causes of conjunctivitis (an eye involvement) under certain conditions. In a study of two African tribes, the Masai and the Kikuyu, it was found that the latter eat a great deal of the grain foods. Deaths from bronchitis and pneumonia in that tribe were 10 times as great as in the Masai. The Kikuyu also had bone deformities, dental caries, lung conditions, anemia and tropical ulcer.

Many persons suffer from gastric irritation due to the large amounts of bran in whole wheat bread. Wheat is the greatest culprit among foods in connection with the causing of allergic effects. Dr. Albert H. Rowe checked on 500 persons with allergies. He found that at least one-third of these allergies were caused by wheat. Bread is a common cause of hives, eczema and migraines. Dr. Alvarez, of the Mayo Clinic, recently said that "according to allergists the commonest cause of migraine is wheat." We recently published information linking starch consumption to hardening of the arteries and heart trouble.

I could go on and on . . . and I haven't mentioned the 7 or 8 harmful chemicals used in the milling and baking of bread, nor the recent work that indicts bread and other starches as a cause of heart attacks.

17. A Controversial Letter from Dr. Royal Lee

All of this is merely a prelude to a copy of a letter a reader sent to me which was addressed to him by Dr. Royal Lee of the Lee Foundation for Nutritional Research. In that letter Dr. Lee states, "While Mr. Rodale

[61]

in general is doing a pretty good job (Thank you), he goes off the beam once in a while (?????) with unwarranted statements. Bread and the grains in general are staple foods (Dr. Lee sells a mill for grinding wheat flour), and animals will stay in perfect health on grain and grass (a cow has 4 stomachs). The grass is alkaline and the grain is acid, and they balance each other. (True.) All vegetables are alkaline and serve the same purpose in the human diet. . . . People who do not get the acid grains soon develop allergies (this is counter to the medical evidence), calcium deficiency reactions, neuritis and various disorders (just the opposite), whereas they remain in perfect health after they get acid foods to balance the alkaline. . . .

". . . It is unwarranted statements like this of Mr. Rodale's which cause the health-food-minded to be branded 'crack-pots,' and he is really helping the synthetic food industries when he makes such statements." (I thought it was just the opposite. The people who attack us as food faddists and crack-pots visualize us as worshipping whole-wheat bread. The whole-wheat loaf is inextricably interwoven with food-faddism, but it has never been proven clinically to be of any value in creating real health.)

Now let us look at Dr. Lee's contention that there must be a balance between the acid and alkaline in our diet. True, there must be some kind of balance between them, but one doesn't have to worry about the exact percentages between the two. One textbook says it should be 80% alkaline and 20% acid. Another ups the alkaline to 85%. A third says, "Nonsense! Forget about this acid-alkaline business." But people *do* differ in their requirements and we can't set definite rations. It is best that we should have some of both categories in our diet.

18. Enough Acid Foods to Fill Dietary Needs

But Dr. Lee speaks as if the grain group is the only acid class of foods. Meats, fish, poultry, eggs, cheese, filberts, walnuts, cranberries, plums and prunes are also acid, so that if one were to eliminate the grain group there remain sufficient acid foods to more than fill one's needs.

One trouble with vegetarianism is the leaning on whole wheat bread to fill the acid gap. But the vegetarian can eat filberts, walnuts, cranberries, plums and prunes. However, there are many vegetarians who eat eggs. George Bernard Shaw did so. This could fill the acid gap quite effectively.

In my own case (I have a heart condition) wheat has an immediate effect, and I am sure this is not an allergy. After a meal that is heavy with bread or cake, I experience severe angina symptoms on my chest. I will eat such food perhaps on my birthday when the pressure from "well-meaning" relatives is too great to resist, but ordinarily I go for months without a slice of bread or a piece of cake.

I want to stress the weight-producing aspect of eating bread. It seems not only to add the weight of the bread consumed but, because it prevents the complete digestion of other foods in the stomach, it adds some of their weight also.

[63]

19. A Wheatless Diet Well Worth Trying

Every once in a while someone will complain of a stomachache, and would never think it could come from over-consumption of bread, cake or pie at a meal. How could it be? Bread is the staff of life. It can be tolerated by very healthy people . . . by persons who have wide arteries, perfectly operating glands, who lead an active outdoor life, and they will write in and tell me how wrong I am about my attitude on eating bread, not realizing that if they avoided this food they could live to 100 instead of a mere 80 or 90. Some of these oldsters are old, but they suffer from various chronic conditions, including the various phases of senility. Who knows? Without bread they might free themselves of all these things.

If you never have gone on a completely wheatless diet it is worth a trial, regardless of whether you are over- or under-weight. Cut out all bread, cakes, pies, gravies in which there is flour, spaghetti, breaded foods, etc. Try it for a month and see what it does for you. But include wheat germ flakes or wheat germ oil perles, or both, in your diet. And increase your fruit and vege-table intake, especially bananas. It will give you a volume type of food and a type of carbohydrate which will be a delight to your system and a great help to it.

[64]

20. Habits With Vitamins

From November, 1952, *Prevention:*

THERE IS no question that the habit of taking vitamins and minerals is going to be with us for a long time, because of the poor quality of the food we get in the markets and because of what we do to that food when it comes into our homes. The vitamin manufacturers are probably safe for a hundred years but if they are good businessmen they will set up a reserve to take care of the day when agriculture will learn how to grow food crops that contain all the vitamins and minerals, and, for the time when the nutritionists in our universities will tell us how we can eat enough of the proper parts of plants and animals that will give us the full range of vitamins and minerals. In that day no one will waste money for vitamins and minerals.

In the meantime we must get some of our vitamins and minerals out of bottles, and we must learn how to adjust ourselves mentally to this condition. We must understand that we takers of vitamins by no stretch of the imagination can be considered hypochondriacs, that the vitamins and minerals that we take are foods, not drugs, and that they are merely restorations of valuable substances which are lost in today's methods of growing and processing our food crops. This is not an attempt at debt rationalizing. An impartial examination into the facts will reveal the unhappy truth of what I have said.

[65]

The first problem we have to deal with is how to answer the friend who sees six bottles of vitamins and minerals on your table and lets off something skeptical about it, sometimes doing it only with his eyes. Here is the way I have answered this type of person on occasion. There are certain peoples in Europe, such as the Bulgarian peasant, who are known to live to extremely old ages, subsisting on only two or three types of food. If they were to come into a modern American kitchen and see the dozens of different boxes, cans and bottles that the average housewife uses, it would be *their* turn to be doubting Thomases. They would really smile at the silly array of condiments, baking powders, manufactured whipping creams, synthetically produced sauces, and many other bottled and canned things that masquerade under the word food.

In the Bulgarian home everything is thrown into one pot and the diet is 90 per cent this wholesome dish which includes a few bones. None of this *bottle* and *can* nonsense for the Bulgarians, many of whom live to be over 100—a far greater percentage than among us Americans.

Here is another angle to the six bottles that our maid automatically brings to our dining room table at each meal. In our case they are merely substitutions for six other bottles that the average household has on its table. We have no salt or pepper shakers, no white sugar bowl, no bottles of ketchup, Worcestershire sauce or mustard. Ketchup usually contains benzoate of soda and mustard, which in carefully controlled experiments have been seen to inflame the lining of the digestive system. No sir! I want none of the condiments or saturatives which disguise and pervert the God-given taste of foods. You can decide for yourself which six bottles are the better. This is a wonderful answer to give to a skeptic and it usually knocks the props right out from under him.

Here is another problem. Some people think it too much trouble to open six bottles at each meal. You can overcome this chore two ways. You can purchase from your druggist tiny bottles that are only large enough to contain the vitamins to be taken at one meal. Filling 15 or 20 of these at one time means that you open a bottle once instead of 15 or 20 times —you can also take one of these little bottles to the office or wherever your job is, or on trips. The second method is to take from only two bottles at each meal, but the entire day's portions, varying the vitamins taken at each meal. I don't care for this idea too much, however, because I believe the digestion benefits more and the assimilation is more effective if the entire range of vitamins is taken at each meal. I have proved this in my own case in connection with a study of my pulse.

One can buy small flat leather carrying cases in drug supply houses which contain a dozen or more of these tiny bottles, usually used by physicians for pills. One of my daughters gave me one as a birthday gift. These are excellent for use when traveling.

A word of caution about preserving the nutritional value of vitamins and minerals. They should be kept in the refrigerator, if possible. I recently visited a friend and noticed that all of his vitamin bottles were on a kitchen table where the sun shone directly upon them. Of course, since the glass of these bottles was brown, the light rays of the sun could not penetrate. But what was the heat doing to them? I touched the bottles and found them to be extremely warm. Such vitamins, in my opinion, have lost most of their value. Have a special stocky square tray, in which the bottles can

[67]

be piled one upon the other and reserve a permanent spot for it in the refrigerator.

Another problem is the changing methods and policies of the vitamin manufacturers. For example, a friend of mine who has been taking a vitamin D and A product made from fish liver oils for years, a famous brand made by one of the largest drug firms, suddenly found after he had taken half the perles in his last bottle, that its label carried a new story. It stated that it was made by chemical formula and nothing was said about fish liver oils. He had purchased it without taking the time to carefully read the label. He immediately threw what remained into the waste paper basket.

21. The Vitamins I Take

MANY PEOPLE HAVE asked me to tell them what vitamins and food supplements *Prevention* magazine recommends. Better yet! I will describe what vitamins and food supplements my wife and I take, and have been taking for many years. And don't get scared at the number of tablets it consists of, because these tablets are not drugs. They are merely food arranged in tablet form.

I will start with the vitamins. I have recently discussed rose hips, the fruit of the rose bush, which is our form of vitamin C. We take about 8 tablets of this a day. Vitamin C helps to prevent colds, and it builds up the health of the skin and membranes throughout the body. It makes the glue that holds the body's cells together. It helps to eliminate poisons from the body. It prevents infections from getting a toehold. So you can see that vitamin C is of major importance.

Second, we take about 4 little capsules of halibut liver oil. This is our source of vitamins A and D, and you can see it is a natural substance, coming from the halibut's liver. It is non-synthetic. It isn't made from coal tar chemicals. It has been found that halibut liver is a much better source of vitamin A than cod liver oil.

Vitamin A is very good for the eyes, preventing night blindness. It contributes to skin health and to the prevention of colds and other infections. It can prevent kidney stones. It is good for natural growth and dental health of children. For people who are too thin it helps to store fat. In laboratory experiments it was found that adding vitamin A to the diet of mice prolonged their life.

Third, our source of vitamin B is desiccated liver tablets, and we take about 9 a day. "Desiccated" means dried, and this form of tablet represents liver that has not been cooked; thus all the enzymes are preserved. Vitamin B does dozens of different things for the body, and I will go into them later on in this series. But the basic thing it does is contribute to the health of the nerves. It also contributes an enormous amount of energy. People who take desiccated liver suffer far less from fatigue.

Some people take various parts of the vitamin B complex in individual pill form. It is thus easy for disproportions to occur in the body between the various parts of this complex. When you take desiccated liver tablets you are getting the whole of the vitamin B complex in the proper balance.

Fourth, another form of the complete vitamin B complex is wheat germ capsules, of which we take about 9 a day. Athletes who take wheat germ find that they have greater endurance. Incidentally, none of these vitamins has any taste, as they are swallowed with water. The halibut liver oil perles and the desiccated liver tablets do not dissolve until they're in the stomach.

Fifth is vitamin E, a natural product made from vegetable oils. I take 12 of these 100-milligram capsules of mixed tocopherols a day. Usually one should take from 2 to 6 of them. Although I have never had a heart attack, I have had a heart condition since childhood, and need 12 vitamin E capsules a day to protect my heart.

Vitamin E oxygenates the arteries and can prevent a death-dealing blood clot to occur there. I am sure it is what is keeping me alive. I am now 63 years old.

This finishes off the vitamins I take. Now let's go into the minerals.

Sixth is bone meal, of which I take 6 tablets a day. This strengthens the bones to prevent fractures, reduces the number of cavities in the teeth to the vanishing point and regulates the pulse.

Seventh is kelp tablets, about 6 a day. Kelp is made of seaweed and is extremely rich in minerals including iodine. Minerals are needed to help the body in all its processes, including digestion.

Eighth is rutin, of which I take 3 a day. Rutin is made from the buckwheat plant and helps to build strong artery walls, thus helping to prevent a stroke.

Ninth is lecithin capsules, of which I take 3 a day. Lecithin is extracted from soy bean oil. It helps to break up cholesterol deposits in the blood and artery walls.

So, to review, I take 4 capsules of halibut liver oil, 8 of rose hip vitamin C, 9 desiccated liver tablets, 9 wheat germ oil capsules, 12 vitamin E, 6 bone meal, 6 kelp, 3 rutin and 3 lecithin, or 60 of the tablets or perles per day.

I can hear people saying, "Mr. Rodale, you take 60 pills a day? Really?" I don't like the word "pills." It sounds like aspirins or tranquilizers or even worse. What we take is all extracted from food. It *is* food. But it must be made up in a form convenient to take. Don't let the shape of it fool you. Its being in a tablet or capsule does not take away from its quality as a food, or as a natural nourishment. It has no relationship whatever to a drug pill that is taken to drive away some symptoms of disease. Our tablets are taken to prevent symptoms of disease from occurring. Do you understand? Fine! So please don't remind me again that I'm taking 60 pills a day.

Regarding our taking so many tablets, we once had a visitor to dinner at our house, and when he saw me dishing out the vitamins from all those bottles, he practically laughed out loud, and we felt embarrassed. But our embarrassment was short-lived because he suddenly took out a small vial, opened it and removed a green pill which he took.

"What's that?" I asked.

"Oh, it's a sulfa pill."

"Oh, a sulfa pill," I repeated. "Do you know that consistent taking of sulfa drugs can affect your kidneys?"

"No," he replied.

I told him that the tablets I took at this meal were building me up. But that one little pill my friend took at each meal was breaking him down.

"But 9 different bottles at each meal," he insisted, still smiling.

I replied, "I have *my* 9 bottles and you have *your* 9 bottles."

[71]

"What do you mean by that?" he put in.

"Well, I will tell you," I replied. "I lead a healthy life. I take vitamins but I eliminate many harmful things from my diet which you take. In your kitchen you have 9 bottles which you'll never find in this house."

"Name one," he said.

"A bottle of mustard! Mustard inflames the lining of the stomach."

"Then my stomach lining must be pretty much inflamed," he said.

"You have other dangerous bottles—sugar and salt bottles, pepper and ketchup bottles, bottles with stuff to make synthetic gravy, worcestershire sauce bottles, and cola bottles."

"I drink three cokes a day" he said.

I replied, "These bottles are what make you take that green little sulfa pill." I gazed at his face that is always broken out, and he laughed.

I eat simply, using no condiments. I want to get the flavor that the good Lord put into the food, and not dump ketchup all over it to mask the poor taste of a lot of our food that is not grown properly on the farms or that is spoiled in the factories.

When my friend left, my wife and I held a conference. We decided not ever again to have our 9 bottles on the table to scare visitors with. We bought a lot of tiny bottles, and in each one we put the 20 tablets to be consumed at each meal. At one sitting we fill enough bottles to last a whole week. We find this much more convenient.

A question often asked is: Isn't the taking of all these vitamins very expensive? The answer is reflected in what a doctor once said: "Health is expensive but disease is even more so."

Paul deKruif, writing in *Reader's Digest* (June,

[72]

1957), stated, "It is objected that an adequate vitamin supercharge is expensive. But think back to the 89 per cent prematurely aged and the thousands since that have gone back to work as the result of vitamins added to nutritious diets. The cost of these chemicals for each person rejuvenated in the Birmingham experiment was *less than the price of a pack of cigarettes a day."*

DeKruif was referring to the epic 20-year project of the famous Dr. Tom D. Spies at Birmingham, Alabama, in which the addition of vitamins brought spectacular effects in people's health, and saved them thousands of dollars in money earned which they would have lost through illness.

Suppose a man came to you and said, "How much would you give me if I can add 10 years to your life?" The answer, of course, would depend on many things, I have often heard people say they don't care to live long. Probably it's because they conceive of old age as a period of senility and suffering. But the *Prevention* system holds out extra years full of health and strength. Suppose you can be sure of 10 or 20 extra years of *that* kind of living. What would it be worth to you? And you can pay for it on the installment plan, because that is what you would be doing as you buy your vitamins and food supplements. Each purchase is an installment payment on a purchase of an extra period of life on this earth. It's better to give it to the vitamin man than to the doctor man.

I take it that a person embarking on the *Prevention* vitamin program, intends to adopt the whole program. This means not using any sugar, or foods that contain sugar. This would mean no soft drinks, ice cream, cake, candy and such things. And that would add up to a big saving to apply against the cost of vitamins.

A friend of mine who began to read *Prevention*

magazine told me that the first thing the family did was to stop eating cake which had cost them eight dollars a week. Quite a saving to apply against the cost of the vitamins!

Then there's the saving from eliminating condiments, those 9 questionable bottles, and from emptying out your medicine chest. No aspirins or other headache remedies, no things for the tummy or for the liver, no alkalizers or acidifiers, no nose-drops or cough mixtures.

A friend of mine with arthritis was paying over thirty dollars a month for drugs and doctor bills. Now she is completely well by having adopted only part of the *Prevention* system.

One reader writes: "My children have had so much of the wonder drugs. One week last winter we spent thirty-four dollars for drugs. Our children were sick all winter. I think it was God's will that I sent for your *Prevention* magazine." End of letter.

If you take bone meal you will save on dental bills. A woman writes me that her family averaged dental costs of a hundred dollars a year. Now it is only routine cleaning of the teeth. The same woman said that in the year and a half since she has been taking the supplements, she had only one doctor visit, compared to at least 6 in the same period of time previously.

What would it be worth to you in cold cash not to get a cold? The amount would vary according to your financial position, but it should be worth something in dollars and cents.

Suppose you fall and break some bones. But suppose you had been taking bone meal which strengthens the bones and prevents fractures. How much would you save in doctors' bills, in time that you are away from work, in loss of efficiency, in the effect on your nerves?

[74]

A few years ago I was walking along a street and saw the following sign on a barber shop window: "Mr. Davis broke his left elbow in a fall on the ice so the barber shop will be closed until he recovers." If that barber had been taking bone meal this fall on the ice would not have broken his left elbow, I am sure, and his income would not have suffered. Experiments showed that when dogs were fed bone meal, their bones resisted fracture.

Suppose you are a smoker, and *Prevention* magazine convinces you that this practice is destructive of good health, and helps you to give up this habit. This one saving alone can take care of all the vitamins and food supplements you must buy. By the way, the taking of large doses of vitamin C can help a person to give up the smoking habit. Smoking uses up vitamin C in the body.

You can cut out the drinking of liquor, if you are a drinker, and save a sizeable amount of money which you can apply against the purchase of vitamins. Incidentally, alcohol uses up vitamin B in the body.

What is it worth to you not to have to wear dentures? I don't wear them, and it would be worth at least a hundred thousand dollars to me not to have to wear them some day in the future.

What is it worth to you never to have to go into a hospital, and rarely to the doctor's office? How much is it worth to you in money to live into a ripe old age, free of senility and disease, having an enthusiastic, active mind? This can be accomplished by practicing the full Prevention system. Vitamins and minerals, and the proper food and exercise can accomplish this miracle for you.

How much is all this worth? I am sure it is a hundred

times more than you will spend for vitamins and minerals.

22. Bone Meal

ABOUT 10 YEARS before we began to publish *Prevention* I began to read health publications in connection with the editing of certain magazines that I have since discontinued. One of the publications I read was the *Journal of the American Dental Association,* which in September, 1943, reported an experiment with bone meal conducted by Dr. S. G. Harootian, a dental surgeon, at the Worcester City Hospital in Massachusetts. This article excited me terrifically. Dr. Harootian was very much aware that with all the milk drinking that is going on in this country, the average person still suffers grievously from cavities in the teeth. He therefore began to look for a calcium substitute, and chose bone meal for trial. Bone meal is made from the calves' bones ground as fine as a powder, and is available either in tablet or powder form.

Dr. Harootian chose 9 patients suffering from major mental disorders at his hospital, because this type of person is slovenly in personal hygiene and suffers from dietary indifference. According to published figures the average caries incidence for their age would be 41. Their figure was 54. All of them displayed a frightful amount of missing teeth, fillings and new carious surfaces.

Over a period of 9 months these persons were given

daily three 5-grain capsules of bone meal, with no other changes in their diet. At the end of the experimental period it was found that in 8 of the patients not one single new cavity formed. The ninth had one new cavity. In one case a rather large cavity was purposely left unfilled, in which food debris accumulated for the entire experimental period, a condition that permitted destructive bacteria to multiply there, yet the dentin or enamel was not undermined. The teeth had grown strong and impervious to any further action of decay.

In his report in the dental journal, Harootian said, "If by so simple an expedient as the addition of bone flour to the dietary, significant increase in the resistance to dental caries can be secured, the boon should be withheld from the general population no longer than is necessary."

Yet, here it is, 22 years later, and neither the dental nor the medical professions have made the slightest effort towards publicizing this boon. Instead, they have gotten behind the movement to fluoridate drinking water, when it is definitely known that this procedure only partly reduces dental decay, and only in children less than 13 years of age. This in spite of the fact that it poses many hidden dangers to the human organism.

In the January, 1944, issue of the *Journal of the American Dental Association,* a dentist from Lincoln, Nebraska, Charles B. Branson, wrote another article recommending bone meal, and censuring the use of fluorides in the drinking supply because of its dangers to the human body. Dr. Branson advised the use of bone meal because the calcium in the bone reduces the possibility of toxic reaction from the fluorine in the bone. He stated, "a calcium accompaniment as a balancing factor for fluorine appears to be a physiologic

[77]

requirement that should not be overlooked when any therapy involving the ingestion of fluorine is contemplated." In bone meal, says Dr. Branson, we have a "veritable storehouse of this element [fluorine] for our use in the safest physiologic form, already accompanied by calcium and phosphorus in a Nature-prescribed combination and balance for a mineral food."

So here were two dentists publishing their recommendations for bone meal in America's most-read dental journal, 22 years ago, and no attention whatever has been paid to them. Was this omission due to the fear that this simple remedy would close 70 or 80 per cent of dentists' offices? Is this why the dental profession rushed to embrace the dubious and dangerous fluoridation of the country's drinking water? People continuously ask, "Why are dentists so avid about this fluoridation. They must be very noble to want to put themselves out of business." Well, my friends, I can tell you, that not one dentist will ever be put out of business on account of fluoridation, but thousands of them would have to shut their offices if every individual took some bone meal every day.

Now, what was the reaction in my own family to the taking of bone meal? My wife and I and our 3 children began to take it, and I can say that cavities almost became a thing of the past, and our dental records will prove it. I would say that there was a reduction of 95 per cent in new cavity formation.

But something we didn't reckon on was the strengthening of our bones which made them resist fracture. Daughter Ruth at 12 had fallen off a bicycle and had suffered a compound fracture of a bone in the wrist. At 25, after having taken bone meal for about 10 or 11 years, she was in an auto accident in which she was thrown 20 feet, and yet did not suffer even a scratch in a bone.

When daughter Nina went up for plastic surgery on her nose, I told the surgeon beforehand to sharpen his knives because he would find Nina's bones quite resistant to them as she had been taking bone meal. He smiled, believing I was pulling his leg. But later he told me this was the most resistant bone he had ever encountered, and the operation had taken twice as long as it should have.

A few years ago, in the middle of the night, waking up from sleep, I lost my footing in the dark, trying to go down the stairs, and fell down a full flight of steps, but the funniest part of it was that I laughed all the way down because I said to myself, "What a wonderful test this will be of the efficacy of the taking of bone meal to prevent fractures," and sure enough, there wasn't a single scratch. I duplicated this experiment one night a few years later, falling down the back stairs which were uncarpeted. I didn't laugh this time as my back kept hitting the hard wood, but nothing happened except a little soreness which took two days to disappear. Can fluoridation accomplish this?

The first inkling I had that the bone meal was helping me was in connection with the sensitivity of a certain tooth of mine to cold water. After a few months on the bone meal regimen this sensitivity vanished. At that time I mentioned this fact to several friends who were visiting us, and among them was a young lad of 18 who said he also had such a sensitive tooth. He began taking bone meal and after a few months *his* tooth also became cured of its sensitivity.

Another pleasant dividend—when I went to the dentist for routine cleaning and he scraped the outside of my teeth with his sharp knife-scrapers, there was practically no pain. Previously this had been very sharp.

A sister of mine once tripped. She did not fall to the ground, recovering her balance in time, but she suffered a twisted ligament which plagued her for years. Once I attempted to get off a moving bus in London. For the moment I overlooked the fact that in England, since autos go on the left side of the street instead of the right, the motion of the left foot hitting the pavement in jumping off would be different than that of the right foot. As a result my foot was given such a severe twist that it lost all power to move. It was completely paralyzed. I waited and soon I could feel life coming back into the foot. In another 3 minutes I was able to walk away as if nothing had ever happened, and there was no aftermath. Evidently bone meal must strengthen the ligaments as well as the bones.

My wife's teeth had always been a problem, being so fragile that parts used to break off from the outside. A wonderful transformation took place with the taking of bone meal. The outside of her teeth became strong, and there were no more cavities. Were it not for bone meal, by this time she would have been wearing dentures, I am sure.

When Ruth went off to college and didn't take bone meal during that 4-year period (she didn't wish to appear abnormal to her classmates) a few cavities developed.

There are several other personal experiences that I would like to relate. I found that the taking of bone meal at each meal kept my pulse from rising too high. You see when a person eats and the process of digestion begins to work, the heart has to pump blood to the stomach, causing the pulse rate to go up. By taking 10 uniform meals, half *with* bone meal and half without, I discovered that without the bone meal my pulse

[80]

rate shot up much higher than when I did take it. On investigating this subject further in medical works, I also found that calcium is a very important factor in regulating the heartbeat.

One more experience: I once went to Europe and overlooked taking my bone meal tablets along. In about two weeks my nose began to bleed. When I got home and began to take the tablets again the nose bleeds stopped. The same thing happened again a few years later in this country.

At another time on a trip to Europe, when a similar lapse occurred, I had a terrible toothache, a thing I had not suffered since I was 12 years of age. I was in Paris at the time and frantically went from one druggist's shop to another until I came upon one who sold a bone product. In a few days the toothache ceased.

At this time, my wife and I, our 3 children and their respective wife and husbands, and our 5 grandchildren —13 persons in all—comprise an island worth watching and studying in comparison with the teeth of the general population. The number of cavities in our group is less than 5 per cent of what it is in other persons of similar ages. Today among our 9 grandchildren, up to 14 years of age, there are only 5 cavities.

In the newspapers one reads various items that indicate a severe general calcium deficiency existing in the population. For example, in Louisville, Kentucky, a man who was attempting to entertain his children by standing on his head broke his neck. Another man just lifts his hand and casually hits the bottom of an open overhead cupboard door, and breaks a bone. A woman merely stumbles and falls and breaks an ankle bone. Old people by the thousands have gentle falls and break their hip bones, which usually leads to their death—and doctors permit these valuable bone meal researches to moulder in the medical archives without prescribing bone meal.

I began to search the medical records for further evidence of the value of bone meal in human nutrition. I came upon a book published in 1938 by E. P. Dutton and Co. called *Fifty Years a Country Doctor,* by William N. MacArtney, M.D., in which this physician describes how often he prescribed bone meal.

He usually prescribed it for the neuralgia of pregnancy and says, "It has been my frequent experience that the patient told me the neuralgia disappeared after taking the first capsule." He states further, "I know what [bone meal] will do in defective dentition. I have treated many cases of delayed union in fracture cases. In no case where the bones were in reasonable opposition have I failed to get sufficient callus formation and an eventual good union."

A Swiss physician, Dr. H. Roth, writing in the *Schweizerische Medizinische Wochenschrift* (Basel, Sept. 30, 1950) describes how remarkable bone meal was in healing the fractured bones of dogs.

Elizabeth M. Martin, M.D., of Canada, writing in the *Canadian Medical Association Journal* of June, 1944, describes her 4 years experience in giving bone meal to children with "growing pains," and also to pregnant women. Of 57 children with growing pains who were given bone meal, there was a complete cure in every case. Of the 56 children with this disease who were given a chemical preparation called dicalcium phosphate, only 22 were cured.

In pregnancy she worked with a group of 25 women who were given 10-grain bone meal capsules three times a day, and 20 women who were given 15-grain wafers of dicalcium phosphate twice a day. None of

[82]

the women on bone meal had any new dental cavities while the others averaged one and two tenths per patient. She stated also that the babies of the "mothers who had been given bone meal had such long, silky hair and such long nails that the phenomenon was remarked upon by the nurses." She added, "We use bone meal in place of any form of calcium for all evidences of calcium deficiency in our patients, including muscular pains and cramps in the legs in both sedentary workers and laborers."

Among the readers of *Prevention* thousands are taking bone meal, and we have had dozens of letters bearing testimony to the wonderful effects it has produced upon them.

But the medical profession gropes along in a morass of disease, not being aware of what is good health, or not valuing it, for if they did, they would by this time have made bone meal a strong ally in coping with the prevention of disease. The doctors and dentists will have much to answer for when some day some Governmental investigation committee examines this situation.

23. No Salt

THE ENTIRE January, 1951, issue of *Prevention* was devoted to the dangers of using table salt. I will list here an abstract of some of the articles. From this point on I never have used the salt shaker, and no salt is used in our cooking.

Here is a statement from my editorial in this issue:

A year ago if you were to have told me that such a simple item in the diet as table salt (sodium chloride) was one of the suspected causes of cancer I might have reacted skeptically, but today after checking the existing medical research and opinion on this point I think there is a good deal to be said for it.

A few years ago I went to St. Petersburg, Florida, and met a woman who had had arthritis. She told me that her doctor had strongly urged upon her a completely salt-free diet and that along with other treatments she was practically completely cured. She also had to drastically and completely eliminate white sugar, and foods that contained it. In the last few years several of my friends who were suffering from high blood pressure were told by their physicians to eliminate all salt from their diet. A few days ago a friend of mine who has heart trouble was told to eliminate salt completely from his diet. When a person has kidney trouble, salt is banned. Another friend who had a paralytic stroke was ordered to eat a salt-free diet. Incidentally, her husband asked the doctor, "Must I wait until I get a stroke to cut out salt or should I follow the same diet as my wife?" The doctor told him to cut it out also, as a preventive measure.

Then are given the views of five medical authorities on the dangers of salt—and its ability to produce cancer. I postulated a theory that for this reason persons with cancer should not go to the seashore. A reader objected and I replied by telling him about Dr. John R. Shaw-Mackenzie who in his book *The Nature and Treatment of Cancer* (1906) said, "In 2 carcinomatous [cancer] patients, their conditions appeared to be aggravated by change to the seaside."

Then there is an article "High Blood Pressure and Salt," which proved that salt is a cause of high blood pressure. Since that time there have been dozens of researchers proving the connection between these two.

Another article was called "Salt Is Not Good for Dropsy." As *Time* magazine said at that time, the cause of dropsy is not water, but sodium (from salt) which prompts the body to hoard water in abnormal amounts —usually as the result of a heart or kidney ailment.

There is an article "Heart Disease and Salt." Several examples are given in the form of medical researches. In heart conditions today the medical profession pretty generally recommends a low salt diet. This is so widely accepted in heart conditions that the Massachusetts Heart Association distributes free to any Massachusetts resident by request of his physician a booklet entitled "The Cook Book for the Low Sodium Diet."

The following is a quotation from the book *Mind and Body: Psychosomatic Medicine* by Flanders Dunbar, M.D., which indicates that salt is a factor in migraine headaches:

"Migraine is only one type of headache, although a common one. It and others are attributed to various physical disturbances. Dr. Max Goldzieher attributes them to pressure inside the cranium caused by an increased flow of water to the tiny blood vessels of this area because of an abnormal retention of salt in the tissues. He was very successful in treating these cases with medication which removed the excess salt, and decreased the irritability of the walls of the blood vessels, and by recommending a salt-free diet."

There follows evidence from medical sources that salt should be proscribed in kidney disease, hives, obesity, sinus condition and pregnancy, followed by an article entitled "Salt a Cause of Deafness and Sinusitis."

Regarding prickly heat, some information was offered last week in the British journal *Lancet* by Drs. G. O. Horn and R. H. Mole of the Royal Infirmary in Edinburgh. Reporting on experiments they had made in Karachi, India, they linked occurrences of prickly heat with the amount of ordinary salt eaten by the affected person. (Many people in the United States and other countries throughout the world swallow salt tablets during the summer to replace body salt lost through perspiration.) Their studies showed, the doctors said, that the rashlike outbreaks could be relieved by cutting down on the salt eaten by the patient while at the same time boosting his water intake.

I would like to give you an experience which one of our staff-members had with hot weather and salt. During last summer in an unusual hot spell he decided to take some salt tablets to see if it would make him more comfortable. His mother did likewise. They purchased a bottle of salt tablets put up by one of the big drug manufacturers and took about seven tablets a day, one at a time, evenly spaced throughout the day, each one accompanied by a glass of water. Toward the end of the week they both became ill, suffering from dizziness and other symptoms.

I never went for these salt tablets in summer. The error possibly arose from the fact that salt must be replaced by steel workers who stand near open-hearth furnaces. Their perspiration salt loss is so great that in extreme heat nurses have to inject them with salt solutions.

Here is an item from this salt issue. "Incidentally, something interesting recently happened about the hard-of-hearing angle and salt that is worth relating here. When I came across the medical article that showed that the eliminating of salt sometimes was a factor in clearing up difficulty in hearing I wrote to a friend of mine who lives in Newark and who is hard-of-hearing, telling him about it. It seems that he immediately began to go easy on salt. I saw him a few weeks later and he told me about his experience. He had not noticed any improvement in his ability to hear, but it had done something for him in another direction. He had been suffering from severe dizzy spells. In fact they had become so bad that several times he had to go home from the office. After about a week on the saltless diet his dizziness completely disappeared.

A few weeks ago I decided to stop using tooth paste. Instead I began to clean my teeth with salt water. After I had used the salt water solution for the first time, the next morning I awoke with a severe soreness in my mouth especially between the teeth and the gums. Years ago I remember having used a salt water solution to clean my teeth and nothing happened, but this time I am much older and my gum tissue may be more delicate. We do know that salt is extremely irritating to open wounds so it may be imagined how it can also be an irritating factor when taken into the body.

Salt Addenda

In the August, 1951, issue we mention a letter received from Mrs. Edythe G. Picard of Hingham, Massachusetts, who wanted additional copies of our issue devoted to salt (January, 1951).

In her case the interest expressed is due to the fact that her husband, who had lost his hearing, complied with her wishes that he adhere to a salt-free diet for just a one-month trial period.

"In 10 days he could hear again," she writes jubilantly in confirmation of the opinion expressed by

[87]

Frank G. Murphy, M.D., in his article, "Salt a Cause of Deafness and Sinusitis," in our issue on salt.

One of our own staff at the time went on a rigorous no-salt diet, and lost 40 pounds of unnatural fluid weight.

24. No Citrus Fruit

THE ENTIRE October, 1951, issue of *Prevention* was devoted to citrus fruit, and the general idea that eating this fruit for health is a grievous fallacy. This I am sure came as a shocking surprise to most of my readers. At any rate, not to eat citrus has become an important plank in the *Prevention* system.

In this issue I stated that "*Prevention* is proud of the fact that this is another 'first' scoop in the field of popular health literature."

I came to learn about the harm that can occur from eating citrus, by reading an article in the *Journal of the American Dental Association* (July, 1950) written by Dr. Henry Hicks, a dentist of Greenwich, Connecticut.

Dr. Hicks stated that the citric acid in the fruit was the culprit. He cites two medical investigators, Stafne and Lovestedt, who found that acid solutions in food could attack the enamel of the teeth.

Quoting Dr. Hicks: "The experience of the present author substantiates the findings of Stafne and Lovestedt. However, their findings, together with those of men such as Miller, McClure, West and Judy, all seem to provide conclusive common evidence that local topical destruction of the tooth material can follow continued ingestion of citrus fruits if consumed in excessive amounts.

"The following reports of clinical cases observed over a period of fifteen years suggest that, besides the local topical destruction of tooth material, there is a possible element of harm to the deeper connective tissues and bony process of the oral cavity, as well as other general systemic evidence of damage.

"Case 1: On September 10, 1932, examination of a white patient, 35 years of age, showed him to have a full complement of 32 teeth in normal occlusion. A proximal inlay was present on the upper right first bicuspid and an occlusal inlay was present on both lower right and left first molars. The oral cavity was not free from calculous deposits, but had been immaculately kept.

"The patient stated that for the past three years or so, he had consumed 8 ounces of orange juice daily between breakfast and lunch, and weekly had consumed several whole oranges with salt, and fruit salad containing orange and grapefruit, as well as green mixed vegetable salads. His diet had been well balanced in regard to protein, carbohydrates and fat.

"The patient complained of a burning sensation of the gingivae, which were markedly swollen, red and puffy and showed no stippling. The gingivae bled profusely on slightest pressure from brushing, touching, or sucking. The teeth were hypersensitive and there was definite sensation on mastication of such material as apple skins and celery. The patient had suffered from hives for approximately the past two years. The teeth were mobile and there was roentgenographic evidence of alveolar resorption.

"*Treatment and Results.* For one month starting September 10, 1932, citrus fruits were eliminated from the diet completely. The patient consumed approximately two quarts of water daily, and large quantities of cabbage, green peppers and other vegetables rich in vitamin C. Apart from this there was no other change in dietary factors. No dental prophylactic treatment was performed during this time.

"By September 25, or at the end of the first two weeks of treatment, all redness, swelling, puffiness and profuse bleeding had disappeared. Other acid fruits and vinegar dressings were then eliminated from the diet and at the end of another month, November 10, 1932, all the oral tissues, hard and soft, had returned to normal and the hypersensitivity had disappeared. The patient then started taking two oranges per week and on the days without oranges taking fresh fruits or stewed fruits. After fifteen years of this regimen, no additional cavities were found and there was no recurrence of the gingival condition. All the teeth were firm and alveolar resorption had stopped. Roentgenograms showed that the alveolar process had regained its normal characteristics.

"Case 2: On June 6, 1946, a white woman, 37 years of age, came to this office for dental care, with the complaint of great sensitivity of the teeth to air and to contact on brushing. She was found to have a full complement of normal, good translucent teeth. The third molars of both sides were absent and there were five inlay restorations in the mouth. Bite, occlusion, and alveoli were normal and the gingivae were pink and firm.

"During the previous six months the patient had been undergoing treatment for asthma by her physician, who had advised her to drink 8 to 16 ounces of citrus fruit juice daily, and it was during this period that her teeth had become hypersensitive. In the upper jaw, all the cervical regions of the anterior teeth and the left bicuspids and molars showed abrasion and denudation of enamel. Several deep, transverse grooves appeared on the labial surfaces of the anterior teeth, so that jacket crown restorations were considered. The gingivae were very red and bled profusely.

"*Treatment and Results.* All citrus fruits, tomato juice and pineapple juice were eliminated from the diet for two months. At the end of two months, September, 1946, all hypersensitivity of the teeth had disappeared, with the result that cervical fillings could be placed without undue discomfort. All gingival redness disappeared and the tissues appeared firm and normal. The patient was then allowed two or three sliced oranges per week, with other sweet fruit on the intervening days, and there was no recurrence of sensitivity. Two years later, on June 3, 1948, there were no additional cavities despite the limited consumption of citrus fruit."

Five other cases are described, all of which benefited in the same way from discontinuing the drinking of orange juice.

Dr. Hicks summarizes as follows:

"Over a period of 15 years, observations were made on patients who habitually drank large quantities of citrus fruit juices. Seven cases, out of more than 50 equally striking ones in the author's records, are reported herein, and seem to show that ingestion of excessive amounts of citrus fruit juices causes many systemic effects as well as local effects on the oral cavity.

"Citrus fruit is an excellent source of vitamin C, which is necessary for connective tissue repairs. Although the ingestion of citrus fruit in moderate amounts as a source of vitamin C in the diet is not to be condemned, it would seem that more than two or three oranges or one grapefruit per week is excessive, in view of the fact that vitamin C is obtainable from other sources.

"The current popular belief that ingestion of large quantities of citrus fruit juices is healthful should be carefully appraised."

We began to search the medical literature to see if we could find other evidence against citrus fruits. Here is a summary which the *Journal of the American Dental Association* (*August,* 1951) printed of an article by Carey D. Miller in the *Journal of Nutrition* for May 10, 1950:

"The effect on rat teeth of the ingestion of grapefruit, mango, pineapple, guava, and the Java plum, and their juices, were studied. For five days rats were fed these materials, to which 10 to 15 per cent sugar was added to increase their palatability. On the sixth day, the rats were killed and the jaws and teeth were studied, using the method of Restarski, Gortner, and McCoy. In all cases, the juices produced greater demonstrable erosion than the corresponding fruit, supporting the postulation that acid fruits have slight erosive effects as compared to the considerable effect of juices made from them. Pineapple juice was the least erosive material and grapefruit juice, guava juice and Java plum juice the most destructive."

Physician Egon V. Ullman, in his book *Sinus Infections and Colds* (Macmillan, 1933) showed that the citric acid from citrus foods precipitates some of the calcium in the body.

An editorial in the *Journal of the American Medical Association* (Feb. 3, 1951) says:

[92]

"Soft drinks, which usually contain a considerable concentration of organic acid, and various acid-sugar combinations, as well as acid fruit juices were all found to produce etching of the enamel and dentine in the teeth of laboratory rats, hamsters, and dogs."

The *Journal of Nutrition,* November 10, 1949, contained an interesting article by C. M. McCay and Lois Will, of Cornell University's Animal Nutrition Department, on the subject of "Erosion of Molar Teeth by Acid Beverages." In their study of the destructive action of fruit juices and cola beverages on the teeth, the authors found that cola drinks were even more corrosive to teeth than lemon, the most acid of fruit juices.

In their experiments with rats the erosion on the teeth produced by the phosphoric acid of the cola beverages was so severe that it could not be graded in the usual manner. The tops of the molars were only slightly above the gum line. In all the periods, the erosion caused by tomato juice was the least (next, of course, to the zero effect of the distilled water), that caused by phosphoric acid (cola drinks) was the greatest, while orange juice fell midway between these two in its potential effects of tooth erosion.

Then follows medical evidence that lemon juice can destroy the teeth.

In a study of various fruit juices on the teeth, Drs. Wynn and Haldi in the *Journal of Nutrition* (April, 1948) produced a table of results which showed the erosive effects of the seven different juices as follows: tomato juice, one degree of erosion; prune juice, one degree of erosion; pineapple juice, two degrees; orange juice, three degrees; apple juice, four degrees; grape juice, four degrees; sweetened grapefruit juice, five degrees.

[93]

Apple and grape juice if diluted with water produced negligible erosion.

The idea of eating oranges and grapefruit is so ingrained in the popular imagination that it takes a great deal of courage to write against them. But I am enlisted in a crusade to encourage better health and must let nothing deter me from presenting facts which I believe will *do* that, regardless what axioms of health it may shatter. In this case I do not advise the complete elimination of oranges and grapefruit from the diet, but they should be reduced drastically. I do suggest the entire elimination of orange or grapefruit *juices*.

When I first read Dr. Hick's article in the *Journal of the American Dental Association,* I immediately cut down on oranges and grapefruit. I was taking large quantities of their juices and I eliminated that entirely. My gums bled occasionally but after a month it stopped completely. I have noticed that when I ate more than a moderate amount of oranges or grapefruit after that, my gums bled again.

While on oranges and grapefruit I noticed I could start my gums bleeding by using a toothpick but after a month off of citrus, even a toothpick would not draw blood.

Again, I must repeat that this is the most unusual health fact I have come across in a lifetime of seeking after health facts. When I think of the amount of citrus fruit I consumed in a quest for health, I wonder what other health information we accept as gospel which is based on error. Like other people I practically worshiped the citrus fruits. I invariably started lunch and dinner with a half a grapefruit and another half for dessert, as I do not eat pie, cake or ice cream.

[94]

25. Readers' Comments

Recently I noted a few comments, in correspondence from readers, about their experience with citrus. Frank Shaw of 135 North Harvey Ave., Oak Park, Illinois, said: "I get cramps following the use of frozen orange juice and frequently from the use of pineapple juice." I regard all canned juices with suspicion.

Here is what another reader said: "For some time I've placed squeezed-out oranges in a corner of the sink before disposing of them. The enamel of the sink in this particular place shows ridges which I believe the citric acid of the oranges caused. For some time I had been drinking two glasses of cool tap water in the morning with a half lemon squeezed in each and noticed that the enamel on the front teeth appeared a little rougher, so I gave up the idea."

A third communication will be found interesting from Luther C. Henry of Ellenton, Florida: "I suffered a physical and nervous breakdown in Illinois, four years ago; and came here to Florida—just to get enough citrus juice. Soon I became worse, and eventually learned that I was allergic to all citrus. Also there were cavities developing in my teeth. I *quit* using all citrus, and began on egg shell dust and bone meal. The cavities ceased to hurt and are apparently healed, for in over two years they have not as yet hurt me. So I know for *us* anyway, lemon juice especially is too acid—and I am sure grapefruit is also. Orange juice may be the least harmful, but I have rejected them all—and am much better."

26. Citrus

A FEW WEEKS AGO my wife and I were taxiing up Third Avenue, New York City, and kidding around with the hacky. I said to him, "Taxi drivers are very interesting to me. They sit and listen to all kinds of people in the back seat, and much brushes off on them even if they are in only a half-receptive mood. Some of it in fact seeps into their subconscious. They become philosophers. I'll bet you meet some interesting people." He was beaming.

"There was this high class doctor . . ."

"How did you know he was a doctor?" I asked.

"He had this medical odor—it filled the whole cab."

I reflected on the occupational smells of people. Once on a train I had sat next to a man who told me he owned race horses, and I could smell that he wasn't lying.

"How did you know this doctor was high class?" I asked.

"I was taking him up to the Harkness Pavilion— that's a very expensive hospital—and when I heard he was a doctor, I figured what could I lose by gettin' a bit of free advice. So I told him about a swelling in my knees and feet and that I had arthritis! And he says to me, 'Arthritis, eh? Then cut out all oranges and grapefruit' . . . and then he adds, 'but don't tell anyone who told this to you.' "

[96]

Now it was the turn of my wife and me to beam from ear to ear, as we looked significantly at each other.

What especially interested me was that when a doctor is not prescribing something complicated, dangerous, and full of side effects he feels like a criminal—because—if the boys at the Harkness Pavilion would find out what a simple remedy he had prescribed, they probably wouldn't refer any more cases to him.

"Did you cut out the oranges and grapefruit?" I asked.

"You bet!" he replied, "and in a few weeks I improved a lot—in fact a very lot!"

While on the subject of citrus, Clifford N. Mackwell, of East Orange, New Jersey, writes, "As a long-time reader of *Prevention* I hope that you don't mind my saying that I get a bit amazed at your constant reference to the etching of teeth by citrus fruits. I subscribe to the saying that one of the great tragedies of life is when a theory is overcome by a fact. And in this case the fact is that for the past 45 years I have consumed at least 6 oranges per day, and for a period of 6 years at a bushel per week, and I still have all my bottom teeth. My upper teeth are half gone due to an impoverished diet as a boy with plenty of sugar plus neglected dentistry." The trouble is that there are differently constituted people. In the study made at Annapolis by the Drs. Belden, it was found that a goodly number of students never got cavities. The doctors narrowed it down to something protective in the persons' saliva. They are probably born that way, and can eat a lot of oranges.

27. Pruritus Ani

Here is another powerful item against the citrus fruits. A few months ago a pharmacist visited me and when I mentioned the medical data I had unearthed against the citrus fruits he told me a most interesting thing about them. He stated that the eating of them produced in him pruritus ani, which is itching rectum. He has proven to his own satisfaction any number of times that he could clear up this condition by not eating citrus fruits. When I mentioned this to a friend of mine who suffered from the same condition he also cut out oranges and grapefruit and within a few days was relieved from all itching.

There are hundreds of thousands of persons suffering from pruritus ani, many of whom are among our readers, and it will be interesting to note whether the discontinuance of the citrus fruits always brings a cure. Readers who try it, please keep me informed.

To obtain vitamin C, tomatoes and many other vegetables are recommended, plus vitamin C tablets from rose hips which will be discussed in due course in this book.

Citrus: Going back to an old note that was misplaced, referring back to 1950, I found that my itching anus was due to orange juice. When I cut out the juice, the condition cleared up. Later the same thing happened to a friend of mine—a violent case cured by eliminating orange juice.

28. Brewer's Yeast

WE NOW COME to the addition of brewer's yeast to the Prevention program, and I will quote from the November, 1951, issue of *Prevention*. The article is a report on experiments that took place at the Sloan-Kettering Institute for Cancer Research in New York City over the course of many years. They were described in the *Journal of Nutrition* (July 10, 1951).

The experiments started in 1937 when scientists found that an artificial coloring substance, a dye known as butter yellow, could produce liver cancer in rats within the dramatically short time of 150 days. Formerly used to color oleomargarine and other butter substitutes with a vegetable origin, this highly poisonous chemical was banned from use in our food industry several years ago. Mixed with rice it proved to be a sure-fire producer of liver cancer in rats who ate it.

To test the effect of brewer's yeast in a cancer-encouraging diet, 3 groups of rats were put on a diet of rice and butter yellow. One group was given 3 per cent brewer's yeast; one group 6 per cent brewer's yeast; and one group 15 per cent brewer's yeast; a control group of 50 animals were fed only rice and butter yellow. Reported on in 1941, this test successfully demonstrated that brewer's yeast prevents liver cancer. *All 50 animals in the control group receiving no yeast had cancerous livers within 150 days. The rats receiving yeast had smooth and practically normal livers.* But it was found that the 15 per cent ration of yeast was necessary to offset the disease. Thirty per cent of those who received 3 per cent of brewer's yeast had completely healthy livers, but 70 per cent had livers with numerous cancer nodules. Of the animals who received 6 per cent brewer's yeast, 40 per cent still had normal livers at the end of the same 150 days, but 30 per cent had developed cirrhosis while another 30 per cent had a few cancer nodules. To summarize: this experiment proved that the inclusion of 15 per cent brewer's yeast in the diet will prevent liver cancer in rats.

In a second experiment dried beef liver was substituted for yeast with similar results. Ten per cent of this food saved animals on the cancer-producing diet. When this protection was cut to 2 per cent, cancer appeared in the livers of the test animals. It seems certain therefore that both yeast and dried beef liver contain substances which, when included in the diet in sufficient quantity, prevent cancer.

The researchers performed many variations of this research and in general it took the larger percentages of brewer's yeast, and dried (desiccated) liver to produce almost complete immunity to cancer of the liver in rats.

Of course, it isn't practical for a person to have his diet consist 15 per cent brewer's yeast. But the addition of desiccated liver and brewer's yeast tablets as food supplements every day could be part of the formula of preventing cancer. Both brewer's yeast and desiccated liver are extremely rich in all the parts of the vitamin B complex, and it could be vitamin B, which is the common factor in these two foods, that makes the cells resistant to going wild.

If this is the case, then one should also take wheat

germ as a supplement every day, for this food also contains a great abundance of vitamin B. In the course of this book I will cover in detail both desiccated liver and wheat germ.

As far as cancer is concerned I would say that if one follows the entire Prevention system, the body's health will be built up, its resistance to outside invaders increased and the health of each cell ensured. A healthy cell does not go haywire.

A physician has referred to cancer as nature's revenge upon man for living artificially. Under the artificial conditions that man labors today he does not get enough vitamin B, and many other important vitamins and minerals. He does not get enough exercise. Many primitive tribes today are almost immune to cancer. The Prevention system is an attempt to be primitive in a refined way.

29. Vitamin A

In the January, 1952, issue of *Prevention* appeared our first article recommending vitamin A in the form of fish liver oils—cod or halibut. But we preferred the latter. In a survey in New York City schools a slight vitamin A deficiency was found among the children; generally speaking this isn't much of a problem in the general population—that is, if we eat a well-rounded diet.

But the Prevention system has been worked out on the basis of taking much more than what are known as the "minimums" so as to produce far better health than the average. Someone has said that health is not merely the absence of disease. This is what we mean when we refer to "the low of the minimum." The minimum will give you a condition short of becoming sick, but what we want is a condition of super physical and mental energy that the minimum can never give you.

In order to be sure of getting sufficient vitamin A, you must take at least 20,000 to 50,000 International Units per day, of either cod or halibut liver capsules.

Vitamin A is supposed to prevent night blindness, and is good for the eyes generally and for the well-being of membranes all over the body. It is necessary for skin health, fighting colds and infections, preventing kidney stones, and growth and dental health in children. It also aids the body in storing fat. But most important of all, experiments with mice show that it can prolong life.

Foods plentiful in vitamin A are: carrots, endive, beef liver, sweet potatoes, water cress and egg yolk.

I am including this little item in this book to indicate that the supplementation of one's diet with extra vitamin A is part of the Prevention system which I have created. I take 75,000 units of A per day. This is one of the few vitamins that become toxic if taken to excess. But you would have to take over 150,000 units to be in danger. Hundreds of thousands of *Prevention* readers have been taking vitamin A with excellent results.

But be sure that the vitamin A you take is in the form of fish liver oils, not the synthetic kind.

30. Desiccated Liver for Energy

ANOTHER PLANK in the Prevention system was created by an article I read in a medical journal. It was a very exciting addition to the system. Here is the article I wrote about it in the April, 1952, issue of *Prevention:*

In the medical publication called *Proceedings of the Society of Experimental Biology and Medicine,* for the month of July, 1951, B. H. Ershoff, M.D., describes a fantastic experiment he performed with rats in order to test an anti-fatigue diet. He had an idea that there is something in liver that might produce energy. He used three groups of rats, feeding them for 12 weeks as much as they wanted of three different diets. The first group ate a basic diet, fortified with nine synthetic and two natural vitamins. The second group ate this same diet, vitamins and all, with a plentiful supply of B complex vitamins added. The third group ate the original fortified diet, but, instead of vitamin B complex, 10 per cent desiccated liver was added to their ration.

Desiccated liver must not be confused with *extract* of liver which is used in the treatment of anemia. Desiccated liver is the *entire* liver of selected, healthy cattle, liver that has been freed of external connective tissue and fat, and dried in a vacuum at a temperature far below the boiling point so as to conserve as much

[103]

of the nutritional content as possible. The final powdered or tableted product is about one-fourth by weight of the fresh, raw liver.

The first group of rats, which were given the ordinary diet, showed the least amount of growth in twelve weeks. The second group, which received the extra B vitamins, experienced a little higher rate of growth in that period. But the third set, which instead of the additional B complex were given the desiccated liver, grew about 15 per cent more than group one.

Then Dr. Ershoff tested his rat subjects for fatigue. They were placed one by one into a drum of water from which they could not climb out. They had to keep swimming or drown. The rats on the original diet, which was well fortified with vitamins, swam for an average of 13.3 minutes before they gave up. The second group of rats, who had the added fortification of the ample B vitamins of brewer's yeast, swam for 13.4 minutes before giving up. Of the last group of rats, three swam for 63, 83, and 87 minutes. The other nine rats of this group, the ones that had the desiccated liver were still swimming vigorously at the end of two hours when the test was terminated. In other words the rats that had received desiccated liver could swim almost ten times as long as the others, without becoming tired.

Here was something to get excited about. Ever since I was a little boy, about every year some enterprising publisher ventured forth with a book on how never to get tired, or how to conserve energy. I used to read them and not only did the reading make me tired but when I ended I was where I started. As far as I could see they rarely offered anything real. They were just *books* as far as I was concerned.

I began to take desiccated liver tablets with remarkable results, and since this time we have received a lot of letters from readers who have benefited greatly in the form of getting additional energy from taking desiccated liver.

One case is interesting. It concerns my friend Curt, an actor-director who claimed to be suffering terribly from fatigue. I recommended desiccated liver. I met him several months later and found that it had not helped him. When I questioned him, however, I found that he had been taking only one tablet a day.

The trouble with a lot of people is that they look upon food supplements as drugs because they come in the form of pills, capsules and tablets. But actually they are foods. I had told Curt to take 9 tablets a day. He began to do this with spectacular results, and now carries the tablets with him wherever he goes.

Desiccated liver is the liver dried, with the water and fiber removed. But the best part of it is that it is raw. Thus all the enzymes are preserved. In cooking, 100 per cent of the enzymes are destroyed.

Desiccated liver is extremely rich in vitamin B, and so are brewer's yeast and wheat germ.

31. Eggs

REGARDING EGGS let us take a walk up Park Avenue in New York City. On this wonderful street from 45th to 96th Street, there are battlemented luxurious apartment houses in which wealthy people live, and it has been discovered that their children rarely get rheumatic fever. But on Park Avenue above 96th Street, where there are nothing but squalid tenements and wretched poverty, rheumatic fever in children is quite common. The same condition was discovered in the slum-ridden stockyard area in Chicago. Investigators recently narrowed the cause down to eggs. The poor children rarely ate them because they were so expensive.

I got this information, strangely, from an article in a British medical journal called *The Lancet,* issue of April 16, 1960. This journal gave another example. In New York City in the wealthy Brearley School for girls, there hadn't been one case of rheumatic fever in 10 years, but among poor children living near the school there were many cases.

To further incriminate lack of eggs as a cause of rheumatic fever, *The British Medical Journal,* issue of April 17, 1954, citing Wallis' theory about egg lack in rheumatic fever, stated that there is less of this disease in the period immediately following Easter when even the poor eat eggs.

The medical investigators were not content merely to depend on trial-and-error observations regarding lack of eggs in the diet as a cause of rheumatic fever. They pinned down the exact factors in the egg that were responsible. They discovered that the blood of patients with rheumatic fever was low in the fats called lecithin and sphingomyelin and that eggs contained an abundance of these two fats.

Now, this piece of medical research does not stand by itself. I would like to refer to another that was described in the *Journal of Allergy,* issue of November, 1956, which proved that egg yolk had a protective effect on arthritis. This experiment was done with guinea pigs and showed that the guinea pigs raised on a diet containing whole eggs powder showed about

½ as much joint swelling as guinea pigs with the same diet minus the egg powder.

What I think is very significant here is that when lecithin was added to the diet of the no-egg guinea pigs it protected them against the swelling of the joints. As you will recall, it was the lecithin in eggs that was one of the factors in preventing rheumatoid arthritis. Incidentally, the taking of lecithin as a food supplement is one of the planks in *Prevention's* program of good health.

I think that eggs are one of the finest of all foods. Medical science calls the egg the number one protein, because it contains the best distribution of all the amino acids. Amino acids are what protein is made of. There are 32 amino acids. Eggs are also very rich in iron.

Another thing I like about the egg is that nature has provided it with a very fine closed package, and no spray poisons or chemical additives can get into it. Remember also that in the egg there is all the food needed to feed the chick that comes out of it. The poultryman never feeds the chick for the first few days. Nature has taken care of that and provided everything the chick needs for a full diet, until the chick is old enough to forage about.

Eggs are very rich in vitamin A, which is a factor in preventing colds. A deficiency of vitamins A and C is usually at the bottom of colds. I personally am extremely dependent on eggs, and if I cut them out for about two weeks, which I have done experimentally on several occasions, I invariably come down with a cold. If you are a cold-catcher, eat eggs. They are the most wonderful of foods. Is it any wonder that an ancient rhymester said about eggs:

Treasure houses wherein lie,
Locked by nature's alchemy,

Flesh and blood and brain and bones.

The question arises, what should a person with a heart condition do about eggs. The average doctor in the case of heart patients usually prescribes about two eggs a week, and some say, no eggs at all, on account of their cholesterol content. I think this is one of the greatest blunders. The heart patient needs the best nutrition he can get, especially in the way of protein. It is needed to prevent deficiencies in the blood, so that it can feed the heart tissues well and keep them in the best of condition.

First, the doctors overlook the fact that the egg contains large amounts of lecithin, which is an antidote to cholesterol. We saw in the Park Avenue research I referred to that it was a deficiency of lecithin in the blood that caused the rheumatoid arthritis, and that it was the correction of this deficiency by the lecithin of the egg that cured this condition. Also, in the experiment with guinea pigs alluded to, the addition of lecithin to their diet protected them against the swelling of their joints. Lecithin is too valuable a substance in food to be disregarded.

Secondly, the latest researches indicate that the cholesterol on the artery walls and in the blood stream does not come directly from the cholesterol in the diet. The latest findings are that the body manufactures its cholesterol from basic substances in the body, and does this to excess when there is something wrong in the body, some disorder of body functioning or metabolism. For example, when there is lack of activity, or little exercise, then more cholesterol is made.

From my observation and in reading medical journals, I believe it is not the cholesterol *per se* that is in the diet, but the total fat that is the culprit. For example, in the average U. S. diet there is about 44 per cent fat. In the average Italian diet there is about 20 per cent fat, and the Italians have less than half the heart deaths than we do. But the Italians exercise more.

So, we must cut our total fat consumption down to 20 per cent. But please let us not do it by cutting out eggs. Let's eliminate milk, butter, cheese, ice cream, the fatty meats and such foods. They don't hold a candle to eggs in their nutritional value. For one thing they don't contain much lecithin.

According to the opinion of a physician, Joseph G. Molnar, M.D., who conducts a syndicated newspaper column, eggs do not contribute to hardening of the arteries. He describes the case of a friend of his, another doctor, who eats eggs every day, and his cholesterol level is lower than when he began to keep a check on it. He states that a scientist he knows in Denver sometimes eats 5 eggs for breakfast, without any untoward results. I have a heart condition myself, although I have never had a heart attack, and have always eaten at least 2 eggs a day. At times, on experiments, I have eaten 7 or 8 eggs a day for weeks, without the slightest effect on my heart.

Eggs contain vitamin B, and the B vitamins are a protection against hardening of the arteries. The field of medical practice is full of fallacies.

While on the subject of eggs it might be a good thing to discuss the taking of the egg raw . . . the eggnog and such things. Cooking, of course, destroys a considerable part of the vitamins and all of the enzymes. Now . . . before we decide whether to eat eggs raw or cooked we must be aware that the white of the egg contains a poisonous substance called Avidin, but that cooking it renders it completely harmless. Years ago, before I knew anything about vitamins and such things, I decided to eat my eggs raw, and within a week or so began to experience a funny dull feeling above the forehead. Today, well-fortified with all my vitamins and following my *Prevention* diet generally, I can get away with it without experiencing this feeling. But in my present diet I do not consume any part of the egg raw.

For a while I used to eat my egg yolks raw and cooked only the egg whites, but we found that to be too much trouble, and to me it smacked a little of hypochondria. A small amount of raw egg white can be taken, but in experiments with guinea pigs, larger amounts of raw egg white produced arthritis.

You might ask, why did nature put avidin in the egg white and thus spoil such a wonderful food? In answering we might speculate. Nature provides ingenious ways to protect the species. Could it be that avidin has been placed in egg white so that animals which prey on eggs will discover that eventually they make them ill, because they consume the egg white raw, and then they will avoid them? Perhaps if there were no substance such as avidin in the egg, birds would have become extinct long ago?

In this case it might be best to compromise . . . that is, cook the egg and lose some of its value, but make it up by taking additional vitamins and minerals.

What is the best way to eat your eggs? Shall they be soft-boiled, poached, scrambled, fried, hard-boiled? If you are trying to reduce weight, it would be best to eat them hard-boiled, because they remain longer in the stomach, thus not bringing back the hunger pangs too soon. I eat my eggs soft-boiled at present.

I am staying away from scrambled or fried eggs because I don't think that people should eat fried foods. There is much evidence that raw oil is extremely healthy, but in experiments with animals it has been shown that cooked oil can cause cancer. This might occur only in weakened individuals and only over a long period of time. It is possible, also, that the *Prevention* system is such a strength to the body that it can resist the cancer-causing effect of consuming cooked oils. In such cases a treat might be called for, occasionally in the form of scrambled or fried eggs, if one needs such a treat. What I am trying to say is that the *Prevention* follower need not be a fanatic, although there are some items in the program regarding which exceptions should not be made, if at all possible.

For a treat I sometimes take my eggs as an onion omelette, using no salt in it. The onions give a superb flavor that takes care of the lack of salt.

Another way to cover up the lack of salt is to combine raw chopped onion with chopped-up hard-boiled eggs. This makes a very tasty dish.

One of our readers advises a kind of omelette which contains no fat. She says, "Cut a large onion into small pieces and put this in the top of a double boiler with one tablespoon of water and let cook until tender enough, then add two lightly beaten eggs. Cook until done. You will find the eggs light and fluffy. In cooking eggs in the top of a double boiler over boiling water you keep them away from all fat. I put a lump of soybean butter in them when I serve them but you do not have to do this."

Soybean butter can be purchased in health food stores.

While the egg contains unusually large amounts of vitamin A, it also contains many other vitamins and minerals. It is richest in vitamin A, but contains also vitamin B, vitamin D and vitamin E. It does not contain vitamin C, which we get from vegetables and fruit, but it is one of the very few foods that contain vitamin D. Eggs also contain iron and the rare mineral copper.

[111]

If you live in the country, you should try to get your eggs from a farmer who lets his hens run with roosters in a barnyard. This insures their getting more minerals and other rare nutritional substances by natural means. The hen that eats earthworms and pecks in manure piles is a much healthier hen than one that is kept in the artificial environment of a poultry house. She gives better eggs.

Then there is the question of storage. The fresher the egg, the better it is for you, quite apart from the fact that it tastes better. A little nutritional value is lost every day it is in storage. Frozen or dried eggs are not to be recommended. The whole egg does not freeze well and the yolk becomes leathery, which indicates a deterioration in its nutritional value.

I also wish to advise against food products that are supposed to contain eggs but either don't or have them in a chemicalized form. Take the headline that appeared in a New York paper in 1957. It said, "Chemists are helping bakers to economize on eggs." But the question is, do those chemists know what they're doing? Do they know anything about nutrition? They suggest that in making prepared dry cake mixes whole eggs be replaced with methyl cellulose and a little extra milk, with, they say, very palatable results. They add that up to half the normal amount of egg whites that may be omitted from prepared dry cake mixes, if these chemicals are used.

Then there's the patent recently issued by the U.S. Patent Office for a process of preparing dried egg white where glucose oxidase and catalase are used. Then an Aliphatic Polyhydric alcohol is used, constituting from 4 to 22 per cent by weight of the finished dried egg white products. One perhaps might not mind alcohol . . . but aliphatic alcohol is a horse of a different color. It is a chemicalized alcohol and has no place in egg whites. And who wants glucose oxidase and catalase in his egg white? Do you know who? The food manufacturer who saves money by practicing these shenanigans.

One more thing about city-bought eggs. Did you know that a hen can lay an egg without a rooster? But it will be an infertile egg. No chick can hatch out of it. It's a sterile egg, and that's what people are eating these days. Today's chickens are raised by factory methods in crowded, unsanitary quarters, where a rooster would create a riot. But fertile eggs contain valuable nutritional substances that infertile eggs do not.

A French medical journal *Compte Rendue Société de Biologie,* reports a research by a Dr. Riboullearo which showed that fertile eggs contain valuable hormones, whereas non-fertile eggs don't contain the slightest trace of such hormones.

In my play "Streets of Confusion" which will be part of the repertoire of my little theatre at 110 E. 59th St., New York, this subject is treated banteringly and I composed a poem about it. Here it is:

Hickety, Pickety is my black hen
Who lays white eggs for gentlemen.
The eggs are not good in a manner of speaking
Because without a rooster (pause) her calcium is
  leaking.

Hickety's eggs are good to eat
Because she's fed on corn and wheat
That are raised on land so rich and black,
But of a rooster there is a lack.

My Hickety's getting so very thin
She refuses to take her vitamin.

[113]

She sits and mopes and lays her egg
But her rooster . . . he's in Winnipeg.

If only Hickety could raise one chick
She'd stop being a maverick
And do her duty like a good hen should
And go back to her maidenhood.

I do not think I shall ever see,
A hen as lovely as a tree.
But this I know and know it well,
My Hickety . . . she's a Jezebel.

P.S. I prefer brown eggs to the white ones that come
from the white leghorn. Those bony breasted varieties
that lay less eggs are to be preferred.

32. Gelatin

In the July, 1939, issue of a magazine I published
called *You Can't Eat That,* I wrote an article called
"For Real Energy Eat Gelatin." I will quote from it:

A real energy-giver has been discovered—plain unflavored gelatin. The discoverer is Dr. George B. Ray,
director of the Department of Physiology and Pharmacology at the Long Island College of Medicine in
Brooklyn. Dr. Ray has for over a year conducted
scientific experiments with six men and four women,
and has found beyond a shadow of doubt that unflavored Knox gelatin actually doubles physical endurance.

[114]

Dr. Ray was given the clue about the energy powers of gelatin by Dr. W. M. Boothby, of the Mayo Clinic. Five years ago Dr. Boothby found that his stamina in playing tennis was increased by a diet containing glycine. Glycine is one of the amino acids found in the human body and is vital to life. Dr. Boothby found moreover that cases of abnormal muscular debility were greatly relieved by giving the patient a diet containing a considerable amount of glycine. Unfortunately, however, it was found that glycine in straight form could not be given because of its tendency to make the taker sick to the stomach.

After studying these and other findings in regard to glycine, Dr. Ray made up his mind to do some experimental work himself on the subject. He fixed up a stationary bicycle, the rear wheel of which revolved when the pedals were operated. Connected to the rear-wheel axle was a pulley connected in turn to an electric generator. The generator was hooked up to a number of electric lamps and a meter to measure the amount of energy each bicycle-rider put into turning the pedals. This accurate scientific mechanism is termed an "ergometer."

Dr. Ray succeeded in getting six men and four women to perform on the ergometer, turning the pedals with all their strength day after day till each reached a point approaching exhaustion. Dr. Ray and his helpers kept accurate records of the amount of work each person could do daily. After thirty days of accurate checking Dr. Ray began feeding the ten ergometer-riders glycine. The result was amazing. Nearly every one of the men more than doubled his output of energy.

Since glycine taken undiluted causes one to become nauseated, Dr. Ray used Knox plain gelatin. Knox plain gelatin contains about twenty-five per cent glycine, and when taken with orange or lemon juice causes not the slightest trace of upset stomach.

The men were given sixty grams (two ounces) of gelatin daily, the women forty-five grams. The glasses of orange and lemon juice, in which the gelatine was served, were well-chilled, so that it was possible to take as much as thirty grams of gelatin in only eight ounces of juice without any discomfort on the part of the taker. Each glass of this gelatin mixture contained the energy one might derive from two-thirds of a pound of steak in addition to the three regular meals a day.

As soon as the men started taking Knox gelatin their energy output skyrocketed. From thirty-seven per cent their energy output went up to two hundred and forty per cent!

Dr. Ray accounted for this amazing jump in energy by explaining that the glycine in gelatin aids the body in building *creatine,* a vital substance which supplies energy for muscular work.

The four women who took part in the experiment were not benefited by taking gelatin. Their output of energy throughout the experiments remained about the same. Dr. Ray explained this seemingly unaccountable phenomenon by revealing the fact that women are unable to store creatine in their bodies. Why women should be unable to do so, scientists have thus far been unable to explain.

It should be noted that the gelatin used in Dr. Ray's experiments was Knox gelatin, plain and unflavored. Gelatin, of the type served for desserts in homes and restaurants, was not used since this form contains very little glycine and several pounds would have to be consumed daily in order to cause any worthwhile change in energy output.

At that time I began to take Knox gelatin and it

[116]

did greatly increase my energy, but after a few months
a persistent dull feeling developed in my head above
my forehead between the eyes. When I stopped the
gelatin the dull feeling went away. Perhaps it may
work for you. For me I deemed it unsafe to continue
with it.

33. Sodium May Be Cause of Trouble

In checking up, I find that gelatin is very high in
sodium and we know, from studying the effects of table
salt (sodium chloride) on the body, that it is the
sodium that does the most harm. I find also in the
Journal of the American Medical Association, November 17, 1951, that a physician who treated a patient
with the amino acid glycine caused the blood pressure
to shoot up from 130 to 230. Over 20 per cent or one-
fifth of gelatin consists of glycine.

I have before me three medical references. One says
that "rats are quite unable to grow when given gelatin
as their sole source of protein." Another says that "animals fed gelatin-supplement diets could not maintain
blood glucose levels." The third one stated that the
feeding of 6 per cent gelatin created an amino acid
imbalance in rats.

The trouble with gelatin is that it does not contain
two of the twenty amino acids of which protein is composed and is defective in two others. Besides, it contains too much glycine and sodium.

[117]

So let us rule out gelatin and go back to that cruel experiment where innocent rats gave up their lives so that the diets of human beings could be improved. Although I feel sorry for the rats, yet men by the millions spill their blood on battlefields so that our homes can be protected from some marauder-like Hitler, whose thinking may be defective, just like gelatin. It may seem cruel to drown rats, although many a kindly disposed householder has often drowned a surplus or superannuated cat without the least compunction, knowing it was for the best interest of man and cat.

The protein of liver contains all of the amino acids and it helped male as well as female rats to keep on swimming for two hours. Liver seems to be the thing that we should have in our diets in an adequate sufficiency to prevent certain nutritional deficiencies. We know that extract of liver cures anemia. No one can question the value of taking liver. There is absolutely nothing harmful about it.

*　　*　　*　　*

34. Natural Foods

The following is from the May, 1952, issue of *Prevention:*

A very graphic illustration of the health-giving value of raw foods came out of the bleak wastes of Labrador many years ago when a famine ravaged that land. A

[118]

famous English doctor who traveled there found a family in which both parents had died of starvation while a three-year-old child had survived. It seems that the family kept till the very last a few chickens to furnish eggs, and they lived right in the house with the people.

The mother peeled the potatoes, throwing the peelings to the chickens. The child crawling on the floor among the chickens ate these raw peelings and thus was enabled to keep alive. The parents who ate only the inside portion of the cooked potatoes died. The child not only secured the minerals that were in the skin, but benefited by absorbing the living element in this food which was not cooked out of it.

Some time ago I met a man who related a case of an old country woman who advised the eating of raw potatoes for the curing of eczema and other skin eruptions. He said that it worked miraculously in one case he knew of. I related this to one of the girls on our office force who had had a severe case of eczema since a child. After a few weeks on the raw potato diet she obtained considerable relief. It did not effect a complete cure but her face showed a remarkable change. She ate one raw potato a day. But I believe she eventually tired of the diet.

In reading a health magazine recently I noticed a statement by an M.D. that "some so-called excellent foods pass through the entire alimentary canal unassailed. Cooked beets is one of these." After eating cooked beets, the red color will invariably show up in the stool, indicating that it was not absorbed in the digestive system. You will find that eating the beets raw will eliminate this red, or show it up in a reduced amount. There is no question that cooking has a powerful effect on the food quality. Take the case of wine.

[119]

Cook it and you cannot get drunk on it. Its potency has been killed.

All I have written thus far is merely a prelude to the main thesis, that a synthetically made product, although of the same apparent formula as a naturally occurring one, is not exactly the same thing. The difference may be only in one ten-thousandth of a per cent, but it is of such significance that it may be the difference between disease or health—life or death. Tell a chemist that a synthetically manufactured chemical is not exactly the same as one obtained from a natural or food source and he will put you down as a food faddist or some kind of quack. To him nitrogen is nitrogen and potash is potash. But there is evidence that there may be tiny "gleams" that throw the chemist's science off center, perhaps by only one ten-thousandth of one per cent, but that is enough at times to get the whole thing out of joint, as I shall soon show you.

Let us take the case of vitamins. It has been discovered that vitamin C consists of six parts of carbon, eight of hydrogen and six of oxygen. Now—vitamin C can be extracted from foods such as citrus or tomatoes, but it can be made much cheaper from coal tar chemicals, and probably 99 per cent of the vitamin C sold in drug stores today is of the synthetic variety. But are the two products the same? Let me give you the answer by citing an experiment reported in the Russian medical journal called *Vitamin Research News* (No. 1, 40, 1946). Mice were fed a deficient diet known to produce scurvy. When it was apparent they were all suffering from this disease, they were divided into two groups and treated with vitamin C which is known to cure scurvy. But one group was given the vitamin produced synthetically while the other had the benefit of vitamin C obtained from a plant. The group that was fed on the natural vitamin C was completely cured within a short time. Those that were treated with the synthetic product were not. The natural vitamin C may have had the benefit of the extra "gleam," the extra one ten-thousandth of one per cent. It was not that carbon was not carbon and hydrogen was not hydrogen—I do not believe that from a natural source one can extract a pure chemical. It will always carry something along with it—the chemist may call it an impurity, but it seems to be a highly desirable addition just the same.

Let us take another case, described in the British publication *Nature*, January 1, 1952. The authors, St. Rusznyak and A. Szent-Gyorgyi, studied a disease involving fragility of the walls of the blood vessels. They treated one group of laboratory animals with peppers, a natural food known to contain large amounts of vitamin C. The second group received synthetic vitamin C. The disease was cured only in the first group of animals. There must be an unknown factor in peppers—the "gleam"—closely associated with its vitamin C and inseparable from it.

A third example came to my attention only a few weeks ago. I was reading a book called *Food and Nutrition,* written by E. W. H. Cruickshank, M.D., originally published in England (in this country Williams and Wilkins published it in 1951). I came across a description of a significant experiment. Three groups of chicks were fed on the same diet. The first group received no vitamin D at all. The second group was given synthetic vitamin D. The third group received a natural vitamin D preparation made from cod liver oil.

The chickens receiving no vitamins gained 259

grams of weight and the synthetic D group gained 346 grams, but those with the benefit of the natural vitamin D gained 399 grams. But here is the most important part of the experiment. In the no-vitamin chicks 60 per cent died. In the synthetic group 50 per cent died. In the natural vitamin D group there was not one death!

The poisonous nature of the synthetic vitamin D sold as viosterol is well established (*Journal of the American Medical Association,* Vol. 130, pp. 1208-1215).

Nutrition Reviews (Vol. 5, pp. 251-253, 1947) in an article called "The Relative Activity of Natural and Synthetic Vitamin E," reported that the *natural* E was three times as potent as the *synthetic* E.

In treating monkeys who were suffering from polio, as described in a publication of the American College of Surgeons, by Charles W. Jungblut, M.D., one group was given synthetic vitamin C, the other a natural product made from citrus fruit. The artificial vitamin cut down the paralysis by only one-half, while the natural product did three times as well. It reduced the paralysis to one-sixth. Dr. Jungblut said that the fruit vitamin may have contained something either not fully removed from the vitamin during extraction, or actually a part of the vitamin, which enhanced the anti-paralysis effect.

Pasteur first discovered that there is a difference in certain compounds that are apparently identical in every other respect. This is their reaction to polarized light, which can be measured on a certain optical instrument. Without fail, if an artificially produced compound throws the light on this machine in one direction, a similar, naturally made compound of the same formula will do it in the other direction. This action is called the "optical activity" of the compound. Now why should there be this difference?

Conant and Blatt, in *The Chemistry of Organic Compounds,* say "the optical activity of many solids is caused by the *nature of the arrangement of the molecules in the crystal* . . . the optical activity of organic compounds *is a property of the molecule itself,* since it is manifested in the liquid state, in solution and as a gas." Two such compounds "are identical in all physical and chemical properties *except their action on polarized light."* Can it be that there is this difference between synthetic vitamins and natural vitamins —a difference in the arrangement of the molecules, due to some unknown substance in the natural vitamin?

So now we see that there may be two factors in the consideration of the difference between synthetic and natural. I have not discussed the dangers of being constantly exposed to the ingestion of coal tar products, but the possibility that it may contribute to causing cancer cannot be ruled out. There is medical evidence on this point that should be studied. Yet scientists every day advise bakers to enrich their bread with synthetically made, coal tar vitamins, and it is through the influence of some of these scientists that many of our states have passed laws making it compulsory to enrich their bread in this manner. By 1949, some 23 states had enacted such legislation. It would be much safer if bread were enriched by the natural brewer's yeast which contains in a natural form all the vitamins that are used today in the synthetic product.

We would do well to stick to Nature and natural methods as much as possible, thus preventing seemingly unimportant errors, or overlooking "gleams." As Milton, the poet, has said, "Accuse not Nature! She hath done her part; do thou but thine."

[123]

I would like to cite Charles Darwin's observation on the delicate actions of Nature in connection with the effect of spinsters on the yield of clover seed. He said that where there is a high population of old maids near clover fields, the yield of clover seed invariably rises, and here is Darwin's reasoning. Old maids keep cats. The cats prowl in the fields and catch field mice. The field mice are enemies of the bumblebees and where the mice population decreases the bumblebees increase and the red-clover flourishes because the bee is an important factor in its pollenation.

But our scientists and chemists do not take such consequential things into consideration. They cause poisons to be sprayed on plants, thus killing off the very bees that could be so influential in aiding the farmer. Thus, today, the yields of clover seed are declining alarmingly.

I must stress the fact that our agriculture is becoming more and more synthetic, and trouble is brewing. But farmers who are operating within the bounds of Nature's laws, who are not using chemical fertilizers and who do not spray poisons are securing higher crop yields. This may sound unbelievable, but so help me it is true!

Every aspect of our daily life is becoming more synthetic, and those who should warn us about it, the scientists, are planning how man will travel to the moon. Wake up, scientists! Get your hands into Nature's soil. Don't be contemptuous of the natural ways. Help your fellowman. Please!

35. Vitamin E and Wheat Germ

It was the Shute brothers, M.D.'s of London, Ontario, Canada, who discovered the remarkable value of vitamin E in the treatment of heart disease, but it was *Prevention* that took hold of it and introduced it on a large scale into the popular health field. I will wager that several millions of persons have been exposed to our teachings on the merit of this product, plus other millions who have learned about it from health food store people, who learned about it from us.

Vitamin E is one of the strongest planks in our program because in this lethargic age there is an alarming reduction in the body's supply of oxygen, and vitamin E has the effect of oxygenation of the tissues. This is a matter of life and death when it comes to the action of the heart.

I first heard of the Shutes' work with vitamin E in 1940 when *Time* magazine was so good as to announce their work and their claims. At that time I was experiencing slight angina chest pains on exertion. I had a heart condition since boyhood, but the doctors evidently didn't want to scare me by telling me. In 1921 Life Extension Institute told me I had a heart murmur, but in the early 1950's I was turned down for life insurance on account of a bad electrocardiogram.

But in 1940 I am sure that the Shutes saved my life,

and I herewith wish to acknowledge my gratefulness to them and to their brave attitude and strong resistance to the whole medical profession, which evidently must have seen economic danger were this vitamin to be widely adopted. They fought the Shutes tooth and nail, with no holds barred, depending on their usual statement, "There is no evidence" when there were mountains of evidence.

At any rate, I bought my first bottle of vitamin E capsules in 1940, which was made by Squibbs, and noted that it was derived from vegetable oils. At that time I was not aware of any distinction between a natural or a synthetic source, but I began by taking 100 milligrams per day (mixed tocopherols) as the bottle stated. And they had a miraculous effect. My angina pains went down quite a bit. The label said to take 100 milligrams daily, or as directed by a physician. I then began to take 200 milligrams a day, and I began to feel a little better. Slowly I raised my daily intake until about 5 years ago it reached 1,200 milligrams a day, and this gave me what I needed to control my angina fully.

Once I went up to the Shutes' clinic in Canada for a full checkup, and Dr. Evan Shute checked upon my daily dosage. However, the Shutes favor the alpha tocopherol form of vitamin E, rather than the mixed tocopherols. I, therefore, began to take the alpha tocopherol and some of my angina pains returned. This may be a personal idiosyncrasy. People should find out for themselves by trial which form is best.

The mixed tocopherols consist of 4 types of tocopherols i.e. alpha, beta, delta and gamma. I get my alpha from the mixed batch. The alpha is about 60% of the total. The less fragmentation I get, the better I like it. Nature mixed the tocopherols together, perhaps for a purpose. At any rate, Dr. Shute told me that for the best effect, the body must be saturated with the vitamin. The only indication against taking large doses of vitamin E is where one has high blood pressure. Then perhaps one shouldn't take more than 300 of the mixed tocopherols.

I have been taking vitamin E now for about 21 years, and I am sure it is keeping me from having a heart attack. Our family has a history of heart disease. My father died of it at age 51, my oldest brother at 51, my next oldest at 62, Joe at 56, Tina at 64 and Sally at 60. In August I will be 71 years old and can walk miles with ease, thanks to my vitamin E, and of course also to my whole *Prevention* program. But without vitamin E I couldn't do it. There is no reason why I can't reach 100 unless I am killed in an accident. I would love to have the last laugh over the insurance company that I will have beat out of so many unearned premiums.

There is one effect of vitamin E that I would like to talk about. It is a non-health effect. I believe it has greatly increased my mental efficiency. There are many persons who are not health-conscious. Under no condition would they ever take a vitamin to make them feel better or live longer. They want none of it. They want to be normal. But if they realized that by taking this vitamin they would be able to get more out of their brains, then perhaps they would take it.

I reiterate that this vitamin should increase mental efficiency, because all the textbooks state that vitamin E is an oxygen conserver—it oxygenates all the miles of veins, arteries, nerves, etc., that go into every part of the body—even into the brain. I can see it in the terrific increase in my mental capacity, which has improved at least 300% since I began taking vitamin E

[127]

in 1940. It shows in the amount of mental work I can do today at age 71. And the future of my mental front looks very bright indeed. I believe that this vitamin will be a potent factor in keeping off doddering senility, which is due more or less to the slowing down of the circulation, the smaller delivery of oxygen to the various avenues and arteries of the body.

From our correspondence we know that thousands have helped themselves to a better heart condition and to other improvements in health by taking vitamin E. Here are a few typical letters:

36. Vitamin E for Thrombophlebitis

A wonderful letter from Forrest J. Caldwell of Illinois tells us of his experience using vitamin E for thrombophlebitis. "I want to thank and praise you for the article on phlebitis and vitamin E. I have been taking vitamin E now for 30 days. My case started with an attack in 1936. My legs were 22 inches around, my entire body increased to half again its normal size up to my ribs. I have had 16 doctors including the Mayo Clinic. My doctor always said if someone could give me a new set of legs I'd be okay. He wanted to tie off the veins. At the Mayo Clinic they wanted to cut in above and below the knee and tie off the veins. I would not permit it.

"After treatment with vitamin E, the blood clots

are gone, my legs are normal. I have no swelling or gangrene signs. I cannot say enough. There are no words to express my gratitude. This is a Godsend. I am 62 years of age and I never felt better in my life, after 30 days of religious treatment with vitamin E."

37. Swollen Ankles Improve

Here is a letter from W. V. A. Franklin of Los Angeles, California, who says: "It was last October that I heard of vitamin E, in *Prevention*, I think. At that time I had swollen ankles and aching legs and knees. I began to take vitamin E. The swollen ankles and aching leg pains disappeared. My shortness of breath, so bad I was obliged to keep my sleeping room wide open, disappeared. Now I can sleep with the house closed up if I want to. My heart beats more constantly than before, when it used to miss every other beat at times."

38. Vitamin E for Hypertension

Another subscriber from San Antonio, Texas, who prefers to remain anonymous, says, "Vitamin E as prescribed by Dr. Shute has reduced my hypertension to normal limits thereby cheating the surgeon out of another statistic!

"I am currently taking 450 milligrams daily and as a result am no longer annoyed with angina pectoris, shortage of breath, extremely high blood pressure and other cardiac disturbances. I have used vitamin E under Dr. Shute's prescribed dosage for the past 15 months. I go up and down stairs easily, walk any distance I desire up hill and down and can perform the run-of-mill chores around the home without any cardiac embarrassment. This was not possible prior to the vitamin E therapy.

"I have had high blood pressure for years as well as angina, and prior to vitamin E treatment experienced 3 attacks of coronary thrombosis. Vitamin E is the best insurance policy I have found and with due regard for my limitations and all attending factors such as proper diet, rest and so forth, I hope to live out my allotted span in wholesome comfort."

39. Vitamin Cures Varicose Veins

Walter Weck, Jr., of Long Branch, New Jersey, recently sent us some information on the wonders of vitamin E. Says he: "One of my wife's friends developed very bad varicose veins early in her second pregnancy and after delivery one leg swelled up with phlebitis. Eventually she submitted to having her veins injected by her doctor and had the usual immediate relief. However, almost immediately after becoming pregnant the third time, the swollen veins reappeared, worse than before! Leg cramps would develop every day late in the afternoon, and she had to be off her feet completely in the evening. We suggested 'E.' Her doctor neither approved nor disapproved, so she tried it. Within 3 days the aching had eased and by the end of the first week of vitamin E, the swollen veins had all but disappeared."

40. A Systolic Condition Relieved

From Mrs. F. Louis Koenig of Milwaukee, Wisconsin, comes the following communication:

"After our local doctors—heart specialists specifically, plus two doctors in the heart clinic at Rochester, Minnesota—had advised me that I would just have to learn to live with a systolic heart condition, I found out about the Shute Institute through an article of yours. I wrote them for information in July, 1953. I began to take vitamin E immediately, and as of January first or thereabouts I no longer have any systoles—in fact, I seem absolutely cured and never felt better in my life. It has been perhaps one of the most amazing experiences of my life, to say nothing of the relief and satisfaction."

41. Vitamin E Benefits Everyone

Another letter on vitamin E and the almost miraculous results obtained from taking it:

"Dear Mr. Rodale: My wife suffered for over a year with severe heart palpitations which would awaken her from a sound sleep at night. The doctor said there was nothing wrong with the heart but still the symptoms continued. Then she tried vitamin E and within a week the palpitations were gone and have stayed gone. She is continuing with the vitamin E nevertheless, because of the benefits to the vascular system. This same vitamin played a strange trick on us; an internal examination a year ago indicated a fibrosed and hardening uterus—probably no more children. Our third child is expected to arrive this summer, very probably thanks to vitamin E.

"My brother-in-law had a slight heart attack which showed some damage to the heart. Since then he has had dizzy spells whenever hard pressed at work, could not stay awake in the evenings and generally was not himself. We suggested vitamin E. Today the dizzy spells are non-existent, his vitality has returned and his wife complains she can't get him to go to bed!

"My mother-in-law had her leg up on a chair most of the summer as a result of phlebitis; the doctor said that was all she could do—just sit and wait. We suggested vitamin E. A week later the swelling was gone. When she ran out of the vitamin E, she gave it a try without, just to see what would happen. Within a few days the leg began to swell again, only to subside once more when she returned to vitamin E."

42. Vitamin E and Heart Disease

Mrs. George Wilson of 1711½ John Avenue, Superior, Wisconsin, writes us about the benefits she received from taking vitamin E. Says she:

"I must mention that through *Prevention* I read of the Drs. Shute in Canada and their work with vitamin E for the heart. As I have an injured heart, I took a trip there last June to have them prescribe for me. They did and I am so glad and happy to say it helped me wonderfully. How the AMA can hold back on recommending it is more than I can understand."

43. Vitamin E Saves Foot

A short but grateful letter from Greenwich, New York, tells us of new hope because of vitamin E. Writes Mrs. Helena T. Roberson, "We find *Prevention* a great help in our lives. My husband has been ailing for a number of years and 6 months ago had an operation from which he is still convalescing. We have used vitamin E for some time and feel it has saved amputation of his foot or feet. So we are grateful for your magazine and all the good things it contains. Keep up the good work."

44. Vitamin E for Leg Ulcers and Psoriasis

Ulcers and vitamin E are the subject of the next letter, from Henry Mosier of Darwin, California. He tells us: "Using your advice I have been able to do more for myself than dozens of doctors in almost as many states have ever done for me. I have been bothered with ulcers on my leg just above the ankle. In 1952 it took several different doctors almost 10 months to heal them. Last fall when they started again in the same place, I dreaded to go through the long endless trips to the doctors.

"Then I read in *Prevention* about a reader who healed leg ulcers with vitamin E. I asked my doctor what he thought of vitamin E. He laughed and said, 'Whoever told you that? It's crazy.' I said, 'You give me a prescription and we'll try it before we operate.' That was Friday and the following Thursday my ulcers were healed and gone.

"My doctor looked at my ankle and rubbed it with

quite some pressure. I asked him whether he agreed now that vitamin E had done the work. He said the vitamin could not have had any connection with it whatsoever.

"My wife had been bothered with psoriasis—sometimes as many as 40 or 50 spots of it. Ten years ago she was in the hospital, and the doctor told her there was no cure for it. For two weeks I have been giving her two vitamin E capsules and one lecithin capsule a day. Today I can hardly believe my eyes. The psoriasis is very nearly gone, and after 35 years of searching and longing for her relief, we have found it. So let us thank you a million times for sending us that card to sign.

"It's been a God's blessing to both of us."

45. Vitamin E Should Be High on Your List

From a Baltimore reader we hear of more good done by vitamin E. Edward W. Jahn writes us:

"I want to commend you for the courageous article that appeared in *Prevention* concerning the proper amount of alpha tocopherol (vitamin E) which should be taken by those who have suffered a coronary, as it seems impossible to obtain accurate information on the subject. . . . Since reading your article, 'This Pace Is Not Killing Us,' I have taking 300 units for approximately 3 years beginning about one year after I suffered the posterior coronary. I feel that I have had a remarkable recovery, and alpha tocopherol is the only medication I have been using since the discontinuance of dicumerol."

Still another reader commented on our vitamin E article. C. R. Disher of Sebring, Florida, writes:

"I followed your suggestion in *Prevention* and bought the medical book on *Alpha Tocopherol (Vitamin E) in Cardiovascular Disease*. I also bought some vitamin E.

"When I read the book I learned plenty, if one can believe what they say. In general I do, as it sounds logical and convincing. Two out of 3 M.D.'s I know who have read the book are more than sympathetic. One doctor has taken vitamin E himself in large doses following a coronary attack some years ago. He recovered and is now back practicing—works hard, too.

"The other doctor has heard of it, read the book and now states that if he ever has a coronary he is going to request vitamin E therapy. I told him the story when I gave him the book to read. He stepped up my consumption from 250 to 400 milligrams per day. He suggests I maintain that rate for 4 months, then drop back to 200 per day.

"I have continued taking wheat germ oil, too. I believe you and your magazine are rendering a great service to mankind, and some day the truth will be accepted by even the most die-hard cynics."

46. Vitamin E for Ulcers

Good news about vitamin E comes from Miss Viola

Lettier of Albany, New York, who writes: "I thought you might be interested in knowing about my case. I suffered for 5 years with an ulcer in the urinary bladder. My doctor gave me silver nitrate treatments, and they helped a little but did not cure.

"Then he heard about vitamin E (at an annual convention for kidney and bladder specialists) and prescribed for me 100 milligrams 3 times a day. Within one week my ulcer pains subsided and I noticed that I was able to breathe better. Inasmuch as I have had no discomfort for about 3 years now, I feel that I am cured."

These are but a small fraction of the letters we have received testifying to the powers of vitamin E, and the medical literature contains many research details as to its worth, but the medical profession in general has closed its eyes to its value. For a long time, in fact, the Food and Drug Administration didn't permit the manufacturers of vitamin E to make any claims as to its need in human nutrition, and it was less than a year ago that it changed its policy on this point. Perhaps sometime soon doctors will prescribe vitamin E more freely.

47. Wheat Germ

Every chance that the vested interests of medicine have to belittle the newer knowledge of nutrition is taken advantage of by them with a fiendish disregard of a sense of fair-dealing. Anyone who advocates the taking of wheat germ or bone meal is classed as a lunatic, or even worse. In an editorial in the *Journal of the American Medical Association* of February 5, 1955, the editor called it a ridiculous fad to take vitamins. "In general," says the editor, "food fads are harmful because they are uneconomical (wheat germ, for example, although nutritious, is far more expensive than other foods of equal nutritional value)." And in the next sentence the editor refers to its advocacy as quackery. In other words, when he runs out of arguments he uses the age-old device of calling names. His last argument is that health foods and vitamin supplements "are a waste of time and money."

How sad! How untrue! How stupid! May I add, "How criminal?" Doesn't this editor really know the truth? Does he actually fear wheat germ? He mentions it as being uneconomical. Was he really thinking how uneconomical it would be for the medical profession if every man, woman and child took heavy doses of wheat germ?

Now hear this: The Associated Press ran a startling item in the newspapers across the country under date of June 13, 1956. It said, "A 23-year-old girl, made almost helpless by a muscle-wasting disease (muscular dystrophy), has been restored to almost normal activity after treatment with wheat germ oil, Dr. Iva Manville of the University of Oregon Medical School reported Tuesday, . . . to the Society for Experimental Biology and Medicine." The news release says further, "There is no known cure for the ailment."

It seems that Dr. Manville had read somewhere about wheat germ oil being able to cure muscular dystrophy that was experimentally produced in rabbits. Now this is a dead give-away. How do they experimentally produce muscular dystrophy in rabbits? By depriving them of vitamin E. Now, if muscular dys-

[138]

trophy can be produced by a nutritional deficiency, then the best way to cure it is through correcting that deficiency.

Wheat germ is very rich in vitamin B and contains tiny amounts of E. Is it possible that people are getting muscular dystrophy because they are eating too many white-bread sandwiches? In white bread the entire wheat germ is removed. Most people cook their vegetables which removes much of the vitamin E.

Dr. Manville's first attempt to cure human muscular dystrophy with wheat germ oil resulted in failure. Later he discovered that the purified wheat germ extract which was successful on the rabbits, for some reason did not work on humans.

Then, "A particular brand of wheat germ oil which supposedly retains natural vitamins and minerals in its makeup was given to the girl." This did the trick!

Now, this is the kind of talk usually attributed to us food-faddist cultists, who say that natural vitamins are more helpful than the synthetic ones, but if cultism will cure muscular dystrophy, what is wrong with it, from the public's viewpoint?

I know what is wrong with it from the doctor's viewpoint—not that of all doctors, but of many. You can get wheat germ without a prescription, and how is the doctor going to live if the public is going to doctor itself successfully? And another thing: if wheat germ has the potency to prevent and cure muscular dystrophy, what else will it prevent—cancer? Heart disease rheumatism? And a dozen other degenerative conditions? Who knows?

It is a question of economics. The doctors must make a good living and if the public does not quickly work out a method of paying doctors other than rewarding them in direct proportion to the presence of disease,

[139]

the real causes of these things will never be "discovered" and the American Medical Association will go on shouting "faddists, quackery, crackpots, and cultism." And all the public will get is drugs, vaccines, palliatives and so forth.

In the meantime, millions are being collected to find the cause of muscular dystrophy, and you will keep on hearing the worn-out phrase, "Cause unknown."

48. Reader's Digest

OCCASIONAL articles in *The Reader's Digest* have vitriolically scorned the necessity of following the *Prevention* line by taking food supplements. But in a recent issue they ran an article taken from the May, 1965, issue of *Popular Science Monthly,* in which Dr. Thomas Kirk Cureton, Jr., advises "middle-aged subjects doing as much as an hour a day endurance exercise to increase their vitamin intake, especially vitamins B and C, and to add a daily ration of wheat germ and wheat germ oil."

Dr. Cureton is Billy Graham's physical health adviser, and according to the article Graham is thriving on his advice, including the taking of wheat germ.

Cureton was the doctor who was attacked by the Federal Trade Commission for having done some research with students at his university with wheat germ showing that it gave the students added energy. The F.T.C. actually brought their action against Ezra Levin of The Viobin Company of Monticello, Illinois, the manufacturer of the wheat germ in question.

The F.T.C. examiner stopped the testimony in the middle and ruled in favor of The Viobin Company when it was discovered that the doctor who was the F.T.C.'s witness had a feud-gripe against Dr. Cureton, that in his experiments paid for by the F.T.C. he had not used the Viobin wheat germ and had used less than Dr. Cureton had in his experiments.

49. The Introduction of Rose Hips

IN EDITING *Organic Gardening,* I came across an interesting piece of information regarding England and rose hips. It seems that in World War I the German submarine fleet had blockaded England, and no citrus fruit was able to come in. To make up for this gap in the nutrition, the government had people scouring the countryside and harvesting the little berries (rose hips) growing on rose bushes, which were extremely rich in vitamin C. As a result the people got sufficient vitamin C in their diets.

As *Prevention* was going along I remembered this incident and wondered how we could make it part of our system's vitamin C requirement. We knew that people wouldn't be able to get rose hips regularly. So I began to gather information on the subject, hoping that publishing it in *Prevention* would lead to the manufacture of some kind of rose hip tablet. This is exactly what has happened. Today millions of people are taking vitamin C in the form of rose hip tablets.

The following is the article which appeared in the July, 1952, issue of *Prevention:*

Olaf E. Stamberg of the Department of Agricultural Chemistry of the University of Idaho has written in detail about the vitamin content of rose hips in *Food Research,* September-October, 1945. Mr. Stamberg tells us that the garden varieties of rose hips are low in vitamin C, but that some varieties of wild roses contain astonishing amounts not only of vitamin C but also of vitamin A. *Rosa rugosa,* for instance, contains from 2275 to 6977 milligrams of vitamin C per hundred grams. Oranges contain only 49 milligrams per hundred grams. *Rosa laxa* displays a vitamin C content of 3000 to 4000 milligrams to every hundred grams, compared to 150 milligrams per hundred grams of green peppers.

In preparing the rose fruit for eating, Mr. Stamberg experimented with different methods of preservation. Rose hips packed in sealed jars and placed in a freezing locker at a temperature of about five degrees below zero were analyzed over a period of six months and showed little loss of vitamin C in that time. Rose hip jam, made very much as any fruit jam is made, showed a high vitamin C content of which very little was lost over six months. But dehydrating the hips caused 80 per cent loss of the vitamin in his experiments. Juice and puree of rose hips, kept in a refrigerator for eight days, lost only a small percentage of its vitamin C content.

"The juice of rose hips in various foods, such as fruit soups, juices, jams and jellies should be valuable," says Mr. Stamberg, "owing to their high vitamin C and carotene [vitamin A] content. Investigations into the culinary aspects of preparing rose hips should lead to many new and interesting ways of utilizing them."

[142]

50. Preparing Rose Hips to Eat

Writing in the *Canadian Journal of Research* for December, 1943, J. Tuba, G. Hunter, M. J. Hutchinson and L. L. Kennedy have lots to say about utensils and methods which will help to save the precious vitamin C in preparing rose hips in the kitchen. Care should be taken that they do not come into contact with any copper utensils, as copper destroys vitamin C on contact. Aluminum utensils also cause a considerable loss. Glass or enamelware vessels preserve the most vitamin C, but be sure that the enamel kettles are not cracked, so that the metal underneath shows through. Wooden spoons should be used and stainless steel knives, lest somewhere an edge of copper might touch the hips. These researchers had good luck with drying rose hips at a temperature of 175 degrees Fahrenheit, retaining 80 per cent of the original vitamin C in their dried rose hips. Storing the dried powder, however, resulted in considerable loss.

They also found that the best time to gather the hips is when they are fully ripe, but not overripe. Rose hips are bright scarlet in color when they are ripe, orange when they are unripe and dark red when they are overripe. Altitude and latitude make a difference in vitamin C content, too, with roses farther north showing more vitamin C than those grown farther

[143]

south, perhaps a kindly provision by nature for people and birds whose vitamin C is used up during long winters and not sufficiently replenished during short growing seasons.

There's one writer who objects to the taste of rose hip products. H. S. Redgrove tells us in *Gardener's Chronicle* for October 25, 1941, that he made some rose hip puree according to directions and found that it tasted like vanilla. There's nothing wrong in this, we guess, except that he had been told it would taste like tomatoes or peaches. He complained of the taste in print and was sent a sample puree prepared by an expert. He admitted that this puree had an aroma and flavor reminiscent of tomatoes, but made into a juice cocktail it lost its flavor and was decidedly unpleasant. Of course some people who live on drugstore lunches and sundaes object to the taste of sunflower seeds! However, Mr. Redgrove agrees that the nutritive value of rose hips should not be wasted and suggests that they be made into food supplements rather than beverages or preserves.

Rose hips have long been a popular delicacy in northern European countries, according to Ivan B. O'Lane writing in the January, 1949, issue of the *Journal of Home Economics*. In Sweden rose hips are carefully gathered and used for soups, tea and puddings. Mr. O'Lane says, "for a soup, the hips are ground and boiled for about 10 minutes, then strained and again brought to a boil, sugared to taste and thickened with four level teaspoons of potato flour which has been prepared with 2 cups of cold water. This *nyponsoppa* [soup] is then served hot or cold with cream and almond cookies or oven-toasted bread. Puddings are prepared by adding a greater amount of potato flour. A few almonds added during the boiling enhance the taste."

51. Vitamin and Mineral Content of Rose Hips

Here are some figures from Sweden showing vitamin and mineral value of rose hips compared to oranges available in Sweden:

	Rose hips	Oranges
Calories	750 per kilogram	480 per kilogram
Protein	1.2%	0.9%
Carbohydrate	17%	11.2%
Phosphorus	.03%	.02%
Calcium	28% more in rose hips	
Iron	25% more in rose hips	
Vitamin A	5000 International units	200 International units
Vitamin C	2000 International units	50 International units

The authors of an article on rose hips in the German medical magazine *Hippokrates* (No. 6, 1942), have as their theme the supreme importance of the relationship of one vitamin to another. For this reason Drs. A. Kuhn and H. Gerhard find that rose hips are superior, for they contain a wide assortment of vitamins in the natural proportions found in nature. In speaking of vitamin C requirements, our researchers remind us that what they mean is natural vitamin C the chemical biocatalyst, in its "nature-given harmony with all other biocatalysts and principal nutrients as nature offers it in plant tissue. The effect of each individual vitamin in nutrition is related to the presence of all other vitamins." (A biocatalyst is a substance that brings about chemical reactions in other substances.)

[145]

Drs. Kuhns and Gerhard found in rose hips considerable amounts of other vitamins as well as A and C.
Their experiments showed the following vitamin content for rose hips, which we have compared to that of
oranges and black currants, two other well-known
vitamin C foods.

52. Vitamin Content of 100 Grams of Rose Hips

		Rose hips	Oranges	Black currants
Vitamin A	....	5 milligrams	.1140 milligrams	.24 milligrams
Vitamin E	....	47 milligrams (in kernel oil)	——	——
Vitamin K	....	100 units	——	——
Vitamin C	....	*500 milligrams	49 milligrams	200 milligrams
Vitamin B$_1$	....	.10 milligrams	.80 milligrams	.30 milligrams
Vitamin B$_2$	....	.007 milligrams	.30 milligrams	1.4 milligrams
Niacin	....	.4 milligrams	.2 milligrams	
Vitamin P	.....	240 to 680 units	490 units	75 units

*Other species have as high as 6000 milligrams of vitamin C per hun-
dred grams.

53. Garlic

In October, 1952, another item added to the Prevention system was garlic in the form of garlic perles. It
is fantastic in its ability to reduce high blood pressure,
it has valuable antiseptic properties, and it is effective
in treating intestinal and artery diseases. In 1938 in
Sweden it was used to prevent polio.

The Babylonians 3000 years B.C. knew of the curative powers of garlic. In the days of the Egyptian empire, King Herod spent the equivalent of nearly two million dollars buying garlic to feed the workers who built the great Cheops pyramid. The Vikings and the Phoenicians, intrepid adventurers, packed garlic in their sea chests when they started on their lengthy sea voyages. The Greek physicians, fathers of present-day medicine, used garlic regularly in their practice and wrote treatises on its effectiveness.

An almost miraculous healing power seems to exist in the garlic bulb. Throughout all these thousands of years it has been used to cure many of the conditions of ill health studied today in our super-scientific laboratories. Garlic, said the Egyptians, the Chinese, the Greeks and the Babylonians, is a cure for the following: intestinal disorders, flatulence, infections of the respiratory system, worms, lice and nits, skin diseases and ulcers, and the symptoms of aging. Until recently the reasons why garlic was potent against these infirmities were not known. In the last 10 to 15 years an enormous new interest in the subject of garlic has resulted in laboratory experiments which almost, but not quite, explain why the evil-smelling little bulb is powerful against so many different disorders. A Russian investigator who concentrated on the healing powers of various plant oils made garlic oil so famous among the medical profession that it is sometimes spoken of as "Russian Penicillin."

Although physicians fifty years ago did not have access to the laboratory methods that can be used today for determining how and why a certain treatment brings about results, yet they were on the right track with garlic. For experiments in modern laboratories show exactly how garlic works in the presence of germs. *Medical Record,* June 4, 1941, carries a story by Emil Weiss, M.D., of Chicago, on a series of experiments on 22 subjects all with a known history of intestinal disorders. These were observed for several weeks before the experiment began and careful notes were taken of everything relating to their digestive processes. Daily specimens of urine and feces were collected. Garlic was then administered to part of the group while the other part took no medication. Headaches, mild diarrhea and other symptoms of intestinal disorder disappeared during the garlic treatment. But, more significant yet, there was a complete change in the intestinal flora of all the subjects who took garlic. Intestinal flora are the bacteria living in the digestive tract. Some of these are beneficial, helping with the digestion of food. Others are harmful, resulting in conditions of putrefaction and ill health. By the end of the garlic treatment, the beneficial bacteria were increasing in all of the cases and the harmful bacteria were decreasing.

T. D. Yanovitch, in the *Comptes Rendus de l'Academie des Sciences de l'USSR* (1945, Vol. XLVIII, No. 7), describes experiments using garlic juice on actual colonies of bacteria. Introducing the bacteria directly into the juice caused the complete cessation of all movement of the bacteria within three minutes. When garlic juice was added to a culture of bacteria, the bacteria were dispersed to the edge of the culture. After two minutes, immobile bacteria began to appear and within ten minutes all activity had ceased. This author notes that dilution of the garlic juice reduced its efficacy and freshly prepared juice was much more effective than juice which had been preserved for several months.

So much research has been done on the subject of

garlic and the treatment for hypertension (high blood pressure) that current articles do not present much actual information on the facts involved, with documentation of how many patients were cured. Rather, these authorities are now disputing exactly how it is that garlic cures hypertension. In a European publication, *Praxis* (July 1, 1948), G. Piotrowski, visiting lecturer and member of the faculty of medicine at the University of Geneva, writes of his experiences with the use of garlic on "about a hundred patients." It is generally agreed by the medical profession that the administration of garlic reduces high blood pressure, but there are two schools of thought as to just how it brings about this result. One group of researchers contends that since garlic is such an effective germ killer, its antiseptic action on the intestines purifies them of all the poisonous substances and putrefaction, and this results in lowered blood pressure.

Dr. Piotrowski however contends that garlic lowers blood pressure by dilating the blood vessels. Although he does not deny the valuable work garlic does in cleansing products of putrefaction from the intestines, he claims that this does not produce a fall in blood pressure. He indicates, too, that it is difficult to conduct experiments with hypertensive patients and equally difficult to interpret the results, for it is generally accepted that hypertension has a wide variety of causes.

It would appear from what we have said so far that Europeans are far ahead of Americans in gathering information about garlic. Garlic has always been more popular outside America. Only within the past 20 years or so has garlic come to have any place even in American diet, whereas, Europeans, especially those in south and central Europe, have used it for centuries.

[149]

An article in the *New York Physician* (Sept., 1937), gives the experience of two New York doctors using garlic products in their practice. David Stein, M.D., and Edward H. Kotin, M.D., tell us that because of its therapeutic value, garlic must contain vitamins A, B, and C, and its C content is probably quite high. The mineral content of garlic, they say, indicates the presence of aluminum, manganese, copper, zinc, sulfur, iron, calcium and chlorine.

Before describing their own experience, the authors review the findings of other researchers on garlic and tell us that garlic has been found useful for many purposes in therapeutics. It is an aid to feeble digestion, because it stimulates gastric juices. It is a fine carminative, which means that it relieves flatulence, dyspepsia and colic. It is an intestinal antiseptic, stimulating the growth of healthful bacteria in the intestine. "Diarrhea from infectious diseases such as diphtheria, scarlet fever and tuberculosis respond favorably to garlic therapy." It is a harmless but potent preventive of pneumonia, diphtheria, typhus and tuberculosis. It is an expectorant, useful in all respiratory infections, but particularly those characterized by a dry, hacking cough—bronchitis, colds and asthma. It is an excellent nerve tonic, effective in cases of neurasthenia and nervous insufficiency. It is an anthelmintic—a destroyer of round and thread worms. It is a rubefacient and counter-irritant which may be applied in compress form for intercostal neuralgia, pleurisy, tuberculosis of the larynx and catarrhal pneumonia.

These two authors give case histories of 12 cases treated by them with garlic. The diagnoses of these patients range from tuberculosis to bronchitis, pharyngitis, shortness of breath, asthma, constipation, flatu-

[150]

lence, heartburn, nervousness, diarrhea, cramps, nausea, vomiting, chills and fever—chest and abdominal cases, they call them. In every case they treated, there was relief, sometimes within a week, always within a month. "In conclusion," say these authors, "we feel that garlic is an excellent medicament, for employment in a diversity of conditions. We believe that the vitamin and mineral factors do much to cause this to be a drug of noteworthy usage."

A reader writes of another use for garlic:

Gentlemen:

I believe my experience with garlic capsules to cure ear canker on my labrador may be of interest to readers of *Prevention* who are dog lovers.

Canker of the ear causes a thick, black discharge which originates in the lower part of the ear. After many trips to the veterinarian at a cost of about sixty dollars there was no improvement. Having read in *Prevention* that no germ can live in garlic juice I opened three capsules, pressed out the juice, then saturated a swab made of a piece of cotton on the end of a toothpick. I wiped the inside of the ear once a day. The fourth day there was no discharge. I continued for four days more, which was a complete cure.

Karl Watson
New Bern, N. C.

54. Olive Oil

The medical profession is always looking for high-powered drugs to reduce cholesterol in spite of the fact that they carry a concealed sting in the form of dangerous side effects. One such product, Mer/29, with the generic name of Triparanol, just had to be taken off the market because it was causing eye cataracts, baldness and skin reactions (*Chemistry and Engineering,* April 23, 1962).

Now comes an article in the *American Journal of Clinical Nutrition,* February, 1962, which indicates that the taking of olive oil can effectively bring down the blood cholesterol. This article states, "It is a well-known fact that the Mediterranean peoples, who are great consumers of olive oil, are generally less affected with atheromatosis (arteriosclerosis or hardening of the arteries) than the Anglo-Saxon."

It draws attention to two groups of people experimentally observed in Zagreb, Yugoslavia, the one consuming animal fats, the other olive oil. It was found that the animal fat group had about 20% more cholesterol than the olive oil group.

The article refers to several other scientific investigations in which olive oil reduced the level of blood cholesterol in people. It then proceeds to describe its own attempt in this field, in France, subsidized by the *Institut National d'Hygiene.* The observations were made on hospital patients suffering from high cholesterol levels. After about 4 months on olive oil, the patients taking as much as they wanted, but no other oil or fat, in the case of ten, the cholesterol level dropped 14.2%. In the case of 7 others, 26%.

Because of this cholesterol reducing ability of olive oil or fat, in the case of ten, the cholesterol level some intrinsic effects of its own, and they speak about the favorable effect of this oil on hepatobiliary function. (The word hepatobiliary means pertaining to the liver and the bile.)

The bile is a fluid secreted by the liver and poured into the intestines. It aids in the production of an alkaline reaction in the intestine, in the emulsification and absorption of fats and in preventing putrefaction. Cholesterol is one of the ingredients of bile. According to these investigators, olive oil increases the secretion and excretion of bile. The action of bile is important. It causes the elimination of poisons by the liver. It is because of this action that olive oil affects the excretion of cholesterol through the bile.

In review of previous mentions of olive oil in this department, it is wonderfully effective in treating stomach ulcers, and Spanish investigators have found that it will protect against overdoses of x-rays. In my own case its use caused some loose teeth to tighten up in my gums.

There have been researches in which corn, safflower oil and sunflower seeds have effected greater reductions in cholesterol, but personally I am continuing with olive oil. Eventually I will probably add safflower oil. But I feel so good!

For a long time we have favored taking olive oil. Everyone can take it without fear of consequences. I take a tablespoonful before each meal. It is especially indicated where there are stomach ulcers, and is I believe, far superior to the milk diet for such purpose.

In this respect I would like to mention an experiment reported in the *Clinical Review Espagnol* (April 15, 1963) in which 6 groups of mice, consisting of 15 males and 15 females each, were placed on diets containing various proportions of olive oil. Then certain amounts of irradiation were administered to these 6 groups, as well as to a group that did not get any olive oil. The irradiation continued for 14 weeks. It was found that the mice that received olive oil were protected against any damage known to be caused by such irradiation. The best results were obtained with a 15 per cent olive oil content in the diet.

Those mice that received no olive oil suffered hair and skin reaction, and damage to the lungs, liver and kidneys.

It seems therefore, that since bonemeal is also known to exert a protective effect against irradiation damage, that before undergoing x-ray, one should take bonemeal and olive oil for a considerable period before the x-ray is taken.

Dentists and Physicians. Please suggest this to your patients.

Harold Levy of Baltimore, Maryland, writes:

"I have a sort of intuitive idea that olive oil is effective against dandruff and other skin conditions, possibly psoriasis.

"Observe the Italians and other latin races who consume great quantities of olive oil. If it is true that these people have lovely, smooth skin then wouldn't it follow that olive oil might be a major factor?

"On this theory, may I suggest that you recommend to your bio-chemist manufacturers the production of an olive oil capsule.

"I, for one, would love to take olive oil in liquid form but I can't go it! However, in capsule form I'd consume great quantities (as I am sure others would). It would be the same to me as taking my vitamins.

"This may be a great boon to many skin-sufferers through the world.

"What do you think?"

I can't go along with you, Mr. Levy, for several reasons. First of all there is a beneficial effect on the gums and mouth tissues from olive oil. But if it is taken in a capsule, this effect will be lost. Secondly, olive oil is a food, not a vitamin, mineral, or food supplement. If we capsulize olive oil we might as well do it with eggs, steaks, carrots, etc.

Let me relate an experience. A few months ago I developed a spot of inflammation in my gums. I had neglected my olive oil for some time, so I decided to take it again. But, not liking its taste too much, I mixed it with grape juice. Nothing happened. When I took the olive oil straight, the inflammation disappeared in two days.

55. A Trick with Olive Oil

Everybody should take some olive oil at every meal, but many don't do so because they don't like the taste. Here is how I take mine. Mix together in one bottle equal parts of safflower, corn, olive and sesame oil. This will more or less mask the taste of the olive oil. Safflower has a great many nutritional advantages, and sesame is to be highly recommended. It has been consumed for centuries in Turkish halvah, but this is usually made with sugar. Sesame is a good source of vitamins, especially vitamins B, E, and F.

Corn oil is included because it is rich in magnesium, but only when it is unrefined. This oil is also a good source of linoleic acid and vitamin E.

56. The Carrot Story

In my series "This Pace Is Not Killing Us," I wrote

an article called "The Story of the Carrot," to show what is taken out of our food before we get it on our table, thus producing deficiencies that are killing people. It is not the so-called fast pace of living. Here is what I wrote in the September 1953 issue of *Prevention:*

The Top Greens

The first thing done is: the green top is cut off and thrown away. It goes into the garbage pail, and eventually is burned up in the city incinerator, fed to pigs or dumped out at sea. What a terrible blunder this is! Nutritionally the green top has far greater value than the pulpy bottom part which grows underground. The greens contain vitamin K, for example, a vitamin which is completely lacking in the carrot itself. Recently, a friend of ours who suffered a heart attack was given injections of vitamin K. If he had been eating raw carrot greens regularly, might its abundant vitamins and minerals have protected his heart? The greens are also rich in magnesium, a lack of which is suspected as a possible cause of cancer.

Storage

Now we come to step number two. In our system of producing food and getting it to the public, some time elapses—more or less. Sometimes this is quite a considerable period. Research indicates that there are substantial vitamin losses caused not only by mere passage of time, but also by such methods of storing as refrigeration, etc. On occasion a batch of carrots come to market with abnormal vitamin losses because of the great length of time they were in storage under poor keeping conditions. Exposure to light will, for example, cause a loss of riboflavin, one of the B vitamins.

The Skin

Many housewives are not aware that by far the largest portion of the minerals resides in the skin and in the area immediately under it. They therefore scrape the skin off, thinking it is better for their health if they do so. They are afraid of a little dirt. A good washing is all that is necessary; the skin itself should be saved. The skins of all vegetables and fruits are the most valuable parts, and account for at least 10 per cent of the total nutritional content.

Soaking

Frequently carrots are soaked in cold water so that they may become more crisp as an appetizer, a procedure regularly recommended by most cookbooks and women's magazines. This causes a loss of natural sugar, all the B vitamins, vitamins C and P and all the minerals except calcium.

Shredding

Shredding carrots for salads causes a 20 per cent loss of the vitamin C and an additional 20 per cent if the salad stands for an hour before eating.

Cooking

The next step is the unpardonable crime of cooking the carrot. Whole boiled carrots will retain 90 per cent of vitamin C and much of the minerals, but slicing before cooking results in destruction of the vitamin C and the niacin portion of the vitamin B complex. Salt in the cooking water lowers the vitamin C retention in sliced or quartered carrots. It also causes mineral loss in the water. Copper utensils will destroy vitamin C. Soda in the water destroys both thiamin (of the vitamin

B) and vitamin C. Boiling carrots can cause loss of 20 to 25 per cent of their thiamin. If carrots are frozen and you thaw them slowly, you lose vitamin C. If you sieve carrots hot, you lose 15 per cent of their vitamin C. If you sieve them cold, the vitamin C loss is five per cent. The poor absorption from cooked carrots is attributed to the fact that the greater part of the cell walls is not destroyed in cooking so the carotene enclosed in the cell walls cannot be absorbed.

Enzyme Loss

Very little is spoken or known about the enzymes which are contained in all living matter. They are important in digestion and in the body's metabolistic processes generally. Nature put them there for a purpose. They are a substance exerted by bacteria or manufactured within the cells. In cooking, all the enzymes are destroyed 100 per cent.

Loss of Cooking Water

In many kitchens the cooking methods are so careless that the water that has drained out of the carrots, a precious essence full of minerals, is recklessly thrown down the sink drain. It is a fact that practically all the potassium is lost in this manner.

Indigestibility

It so happens that the carrot is somewhat fibrous. Some of it resists mastication, and no matter how much you chew it, that portion can do nothing for the human body. So we must chalk up another loss.

Effect of Chemical Fertilizer

We must not overlook the nutritional effect on the

carrot of the large amount of chemical fertilizers used in growing them under the artificial conditions of to-day's agriculture. A carrot grown in 1870, for example, was far different from the average one grown today. The present-day carrot has less vitamins and minerals, and you can prove this in no time by feeding two groups of rabbits—one with carrots grown with chemical fertilizers—the other with carrots grown with organic matter such as manure, leaves, weeds, etc. To this extent, therefore, there was that much less need in 1870 to take vitamins.

Use of Added Sugar

Many housewives douse practically everything they cook or handle in the kitchen with sugar, and the carrot does not escape. In such cases one does not taste carrot, but sugar. However, sugar, in addition to its other bad habits, neutralizes the calcium with which it comes in contact, and when one considers that the government found in a recent survey that 85 per cent of the public is calcium deficient, one can see, in the addition of so much sugar to our foods, one of the reasons for that deficiency.

The Garbage Pail

It is not enough that man destroys so much of the nutritional percentage of the carrot; he is not yet satis-fied. At the last moment he decides not to eat it all and leaves a small portion, sometimes not so small, to find its way into the garbage pail and to the city inciner-ator where it is burned up.

Conclusion

What is left is a painfully pitiful portion of what the carrot had to offer to start with. Yet when we eat a dish

[159]

of cooked carrots we usually do it with a glow of satisfaction—with a feeling that we are eating something that will fortify us against come what may in the battle for health. Is it any wonder then that the executives of large companies are dropping dead every day from heart disease? It is sad to note that nutritionists have eyes but cannot see that *they* are the ones who could set things right by recognizing conditions for what they are and coming out in a tremendous campaign recommending the taking of vitamins and minerals by every man, woman and child.

It is not the so-called fast pace that is killing people, but a degenerating and weakening of the body due to an emasculation of its food. It is not only the carrot—when one sees what is being done to our bread, milk, and other foods, a case is built for the increasing deaths not only from heart disease but also from cancer, polio and the host of other degenerative diseases which are multiplying at such an alarming rate.

The next time some doctor or friend tells you that you should eat your vitamins with a knife and a fork, tell him the story of the carrot and see what he says then. We *must* take vitamins if we wish to be healthy and the nation as a whole must do it, or God alone knows what will happen to the second or third generation coming up—generations inheriting weaknesses passed on to them by us, generations which few of us will live to see unless we augment our diet with vitamins and minerals.

57. Softened Water

As my experience accumulated in the field of preventing sickness, I became somewhat of a compiler. We searched the medical journals. At the beginning I did much of this myself. Later we developed a staff that did a more thorough job of it.

I received long lists of articles the staff thought would interest me. Here and there appeared nuggets upon which I pounced. As the years passed I wrote articles based on compiled medical information which helped develop the Prevention system.

At this moment I would like to discuss something I found in *Consumers' Research Bulletin* (Feb., 1953) which I made much use of in later years. I wrote about it in *Prevention,* June, 1953, as follows:

Consumers' Research Bulletin reminds us that the sodium content of softened water is high and that high-sodium water is very undesirable in many cases of heart trouble, especially in older people, where the sodium collects in the body, attracts water to itself and brings about overweight or edema (swelling), both of which increase the work of an already overloaded heart. In addition, says the *Bulletin,* "scientific studies have established a relationship unfavorable to the use of soft water for drinking and cooking and have shown that when the drinking water is soft there is a marked tendency toward increased deficiencies in tooth and bone formation and increased tooth decay. In general, if a water-softening system is installed in a home, it will be advisable to provide a cold-water tap through which water that has not been softened is supplied for drinking and cooking."

I started a campaign in *Prevention* to advise people to take the water softening device off the cold water faucet. This can be done quite easily. It is our opinion that one should not drink water that has been softened by home-type water softener outfits, because such water has had much of its calcium and magnesium removed and replaced by sodium. Sodium is known to cause high blood pressure, and to be detrimental to the heart. The drinking of artificially softened water must have killed hundreds of thousands of heart patients long before their time.

Here is an item from our *Health Bulletin*, April 25, 1964: "The high natural sodium content of certain water supplies caused a recurrence of congestive heart disease in two patients, a Public Health Service nutrition consultant told the Ohio Dietetic Association last week. The Public Health Service is continuing its nationwide study of the salt content of water."

It should also make a nationwide study of how drinking artificially softened water affects the human heart. It should suggest that people have water softening devices attached only to the hot water faucet. This will provide all the softening needed for bathing, laundering, etc.

Never drink artificially softened water!

Here is an item I wrote in *Prevention*, August 1963:

According to the Medical Tribune (May 13, 1963), the U. S. Public Health Service plans to analyze drinking water from about 3,000 communities for sodium content. This study is aimed at helping heart specialists to maintain their patients on a low-salt (sodium chloride) diet. Physicians "may be unaware of the

[162]

amount of sodium reaching the patient through drinking water or cooking."

There is another source of sodium contamination in water that the Public Health Service is overlooking, and this source may give far more sodium than that contained naturally in drinking water. I am referring to the sodium placed in water in order to soften it. Water softening devices work by withdrawing calcium and magnesium from water, these elements being the cause of the water's hardness. This is done by a chemical action in which sodium is exchanged for the calcium and magnesium.

It is suggested, therefore, that only the hot water of a home be softened. I am wondering how many millions of heart attacks have been caused by susceptible people drinking artificially softened water. Where are our doctors?

Here is another item—November, 1963, *Prevention:*

Ventura County, California, has a law banning water softener equipment in homes. This law has been in existence for three years, but it is known that bootlegging is going on. For many years, I have been advising against softening the water on the cold water faucet, because in softening water, the hardening element, calcium (lime), is removed by the addition of sodium, which is not only dangerous for heart and high blood pressure cases, but could also produce these conditions in susceptible people.

It is this same sodium that the Ventura County supervisors fear will contaminate the underground water. The supervisors are not worrying about the danger to people drinking such sodium-containing water. They are concerned mainly about its effect on agriculture because, in irrigation, it is the underground water that is drawn upon.

[163]

Again, may I caution people who use water softeners: an adequate effect can be produced by softening the hot water only. It is extremely dangerous to drink artificially softened water. In fact, medical statistics prove that even in regions where the water is naturally soft, there are more heart cases than where the drinking water is hard.

In closing this chapter may I mention the case of Doris Grant, a well-known health writer in England, who wrote me that I had saved her life. She had been very ill with a long list of terrible symptoms which had her doctors baffled. Nothing could be done for her.

Then she read my article about artificially softened water. She removed the softening apparatus from the cold water faucet, and in a few weeks all her symptoms left her.

Here is an excerpt from a letter written to us by Mrs. William F. Schrock, Jr., of Santa Barbara, Calif.:

"For awhile, after drinking artificially softened water I suffered severe intestinal distress, at the same time coincidentally that soft water was connected to my cold water tap. A month before this was removed, I had symptoms of a possible heart attack, according to my local chiropractor, a Dr. Richard Van Rumpt, founder and director of non-force technic in Chiropractic. I went to my local M.D. telling him of chest pains, and arm pains which he indicated were symptoms, but at the time of his diagnosis stated there was no sign of heart disease at that moment. When the soft water service was changed only to the hot water tap, the diarrhea promptly stopped."

[164]

58. Chlorine—The Forgotten Chemical

IN THE EXCITEMENT and the unholy zeal to railroad through fluoridation of our drinking waters, people seem to have forgotten all about the fact that our water is being chlorinated. They take chlorine for granted. It is a *fait accompli,* and they believe that nothing can be done about it. Chlorination has been in use for so long that time has given it a sort of complacent acceptance. The sad part of it is, however, that in the eyes of some people it has a halo. The best people are for it, aren't they? The schools, and doctors and congressmen recommend it, do they not? After all, we've been drinking chlorinated water all our lives and we aren't dead yet, so it couldn't possibly be harmful.

I have heard dentists, in public recommendations of the use of fluorine, practically predicate their entire case on the fact that since a city has the right to place chlorine in the water, it may also, therefore, put in fluorine. But fluorine is used to reduce cavities in the teeth of children—while chlorination is resorted to, to kill harmful bacteria that can cause diseases like typhoid. The latter has the barest semblance of justification, but the use of fluorine would set off a new dangerous trend. Where would municipalities stop? Would they eventually put aspirin in the water to prevent headaches?

[165]

59. A Potent Poison

Chlorine is a powerful disinfectant—a potent poison, highly irritative to the skin and the mucous membranes. In Clorox it is used for bleaching, and it has a great many industrial uses because of its active nature as a chemical element. If house-plants are watered with chlorinated water they will not thrive, nor will guppies live in such water. Many years ago, I was told by a man who conducted a market where fish were kept alive till sold, that the day the waterworks placed a charge of chlorine into the water, all his fish died.

Physicians do not seem to be aware, nor do they care much about the effect of chlorine on the human body. One rarely sees references to it in medical literature. In his book *How To Help Your Doctor Help You* (Dell), Walter C. Alvarez, M.D. says: "It is hard to explain why many a highly sensitive person reacts strongly and in an allergic way to such simple chemical substances as aspirin or sugar or chlorine in the city water. These small molecules are very different from the huge and extremely complicated molecules of protein which were originally supposed to produce all allergic reactions."

60. Physiological Reaction

In the *Journal of Allergy* for November 1944, appears an article in which M. J. Gutmann, M.D., of Jerusalem writes of a case of giant hives in an English officer. Skin tests showed no evidence of sensitivity; testing with over 40 different food substances showed no allergy nor were there any indications of bacterial allergy.

Yet this officer's hives disappeared when he was transferred from Jerusalem to other stations. He could recollect no difference in his diet and way of life at these other stations except he drank mineral waters. As soon as he returned to Jerusalem and once again drank the city water, he developed hives immediately. The water in Jerusalem is chlorinated. When chlorinated water is heated, for coffee, tea and so forth, the chlorine is given off into the air and can produce no symptoms. But, for those who drink the water cold, out of the faucet, a number of symptoms may arise.

Dr. Gutmann reviews an article in the *Journal of Allergy* for 1934 in which chlorine in water was found to be the cause of asthma and functional colitis. When the patient was put on distilled water exclusively for three days, he experienced no return of either disorder. Then when one drop of sodium hypochlorite was placed in his drinking water, his asthma and colitis promptly returned. Dr. Gutmann tells us that he has had other patients who got hives from the addition of even the smallest amounts of chlorine to their drinking water.

[167]

One was a woman of 28 who had hives from childhood. All her life she had tried the most extreme kinds
of diet in an effort to locate the food which was causing the allergy. Eventually someone thought of changing her drinking water. The hives disappeared within
a few days. As soon as she returned to chlorinated
drinking water, the eruptions appeared within a short
time.

61. Safety Never Proved

One day I was reading the *Journal of the American
Medical Association* (July 28, 1951 issue) and I saw
something that astounded me. In the section where the
doctors ask questions, there appeared a question to the
editor which asked whether studies had ever been made
to determine the harmful effects of chlorinated water
used for drinking purposes. The editor's answer said
that a careful check of all the literature and all available information revealed the fact that no organized
investigation had ever been made of the effect of
chlorine on the human body. He admitted that there
had been cases of allergic skin inflammation and many
outbreaks of asthma that were traced to chlorine, but
the editor refers to them as allergies.

In *Bridges' Dietetics for the Clinician* by Harry J.
Johnson, M.D. (1949, Lea and Febiger) on page 91
appears the statement that chlorine destroys vitamin E.

Another medical bit of evidence incriminating
chlorine is contained in a book called *Poisoning* by W.

F. von Oettingen, M.D., page 72 (Paul Hoebner, Inc.). The author says, "It has been claimed that injury of the mitral valve (of the heart) and cardiac (heart) insufficiency may result from severe exposure to chlorine, or carbon monoxide. Coronary thrombosis, characterized by palpitation, irregularities of the heart beat, and anxiety, has been reported in poisoning with chlorine, carbon monoxide and ferric chloride." The latter is a chlorine compound.

62. Pure Water Possible

When I was in the small town of Appeldoorn in Holland I was amazed to discover that the people there drank the water without a single chemical being put into it for any purpose whatever. Upon investigation I found that the drinking water of this town of about 30,000 people is obtained from deep wells sunk for the purpose. This would seem to be an ideal solution for many American cities. The existing water lines could be maintained for non-drinking and industrial purposes, and a separate line could be used merely for drinking water.

As far as chlorination is concerned, have we re-evaluated the need for it based on the fact that the general conception of sanitation has improved so much today compared to the primitive conditions of 1900? We are treating our water based on a 1900 diagnosis. Is it not time for the medical profession to take another look?

We must keep our drinking water sources unpolluted.

If we study methods to keep water as clean as possible, then chlorination, or any other chemicalization would not be required. There must be safer means. The Romans used silver to purify their water—infinitesimal amounts of it, and I have heard that some city in this country is experimenting with it. Water can also be purified by ultraviolet light. Perhaps the cities could pasteurize the water as it goes into the mains, that is, to boil it in order to kill offensive organisms. Incidentally, this may be an excellent idea for the home. Boil all chlorinated water to be used for drinking, because boiling will eliminate all traces of chlorine from it. It will not, however, get rid of the fluorine. Distillation will do that. But cities might rig up automatic pasteurizing equipment that could work economically. Where are our vaunted engineering brains? You don't see them putting chlorine in milk to kill organisms. No! Milk is a commercial product that brings dollars. But water? What care the politicians if it reeks of chlorine!

What we need is pure water societies to spring up all over the United States, which could eventually grow into general health groups that could wield great power in moulding public and official opinion on health matters.

In the meantime, either boil your drinking water or buy bottled spring water, and watch carefully to observe the effects on the health of the family.

63. Minerals in Water

I HAD A LESSON recently in what the taste of water signifies. I was in a prominent restaurant in Allentown, and the water tasted horribly of chlorine. I commented on this to our waitress, and she brought us some distilled water from the bar. It seems that when it comes to drinking alcoholic beverages, the taste of chlorine would spoil the effect! So they use distilled water in the cocktails!

But when I drank that distilled water I found it to be completely devoid of any taste. It was as neutral a substance as I had ever tasted. I did not enjoy it! This made me think. In distilling water, all the minerals are removed. So it is the minerals that give the taste to water. And this is what makes purchased spring water so tasty. They evidently use springs in which the water abounds in minerals.

Now, the question is, does this apply to solid foods also? When one carrot tastes better than another, is this because it contains more minerals? Organic gardeners have found that organically raised food tastes better than food raised with chemical fertilizers. Perhaps this may be because the organically raised food is much richer in minerals.

Take the eggs on our organically run farm. How wonderful they taste! And now we may have the reason. Minerals!

Talking about the taste of water reminds me of the old lady a long time ago in London who drank Thames River water. When they installed a filtering system, and she drank her first glass of the filtered water, she spit it out. "Phew," she said. "This water has no taste!"

Many chemicals are used at water works, one purpose of which is to make water more palatable. *Newsweek* (Dec. 2, 1963) said, "No less than 25 chemicals are routinely used to make municipal water supplies safe and palatable." Certain algae, for example, give a peculiar taste to water and they must be destroyed.

[171]

Copper sulfate is usually used for this purpose, but lately it has been discovered that an excess of copper causes fatty plaques to form on the blood-vessel walls. What confusion! The one who does one thing in our complicated civilization does not know the full effect of what he is doing. After all, the water works engineer is not a doctor, neither is the doctor a water works engineer. So a heart patient drinks copperized water, including the effect of copper from his household copper water pipes. Then comes a heart attack, and the doctors shrug their shoulders: "We don't know what could be the cause!"

64. Coffee and Tea

THIS IS BEING written by someone who has been drinking coffee practically since infancy, so you might say that he is slightly prejudiced, and you would be right if you said that. On the other hand, this person is wonderfully health-conscious in practically every other respect. Now, before I proceed with my rationalization and justifications, may I tell you a little story. Once there was a sculptor who was carving out a statue and it was a marvelous piece of work—perfect in every detail. As he worked, his friends came to admire. The statue he was working on became the talk of the town and everyone agreed that it would be the crowning achievement of this man. On the last day, however, the sculptor made a tiny nick on the figure in a fairly prominent spot and a friend who happened to be there at the time asked him why he did it. The artist's reply was, "Only the gods are perfect. I did this so that the gods would not be jealous."

In my own case I am building up a very strong and healthy body. I take no sugar in any form, excluding from my diet candies, cakes, ice creams, sodas and so forth, except for an occasional slight deviation. I am on a low salt diet. I am keeping my weight down. I do not smoke nor drink alcoholic liquors. I take liberally of natural vitamins and minerals. We have our own farm and about 80 per cent of our food is raised there, including meat (steers, sheep and poultry). These crops are grown by the organic method—without chemical fertilizers or poisonous insecticides and a lot of them are consumed fresh with no long periods of storage and losses of nutritional content. All of this has gradually given me an immunity to headaches, colds and disease in general.

So I drink coffee! Now on with my story! I know that I would have been better off if I had never started with coffee. The body was not made to need it and, no doubt, could do a much better job without it. But since I did not receive the proper guidance when I was young, I must face my problem in the most intelligent manner possible. Let us always try to use our sense of intelligence, not our emotions, in resolving life's problems.

The question is, will the body function better without coffee after a lifetime of using it? My experience indicates a negative answer in my own case.

Up to the age of about 53 I was satisfied with three cups of coffee a day, but when I began to go to Europe I came back a six-cup-a-day man. It is difficult to resist it in England and especially in Germany if you visit

[173]

with the natives. They drink a lot of tea and coffee respectively.

I have had a heart condition ever since I was about twenty or so. At least at that time I was told that I had a heart murmur, but I believe that all was not well with my ticker perhaps since birth. I understand that in our glorious country today twenty-five to fifty thousand babies are born each year with heart trouble. At any rate, as a boy, I never could swim more than eight or ten strokes without having to give up, due to shortness of breath.

At twenty I began to play tennis and overdid it, thus no doubt, bringing on the heart murmur. But I am sure that if my heart had been basically sound, in the beginning, the tennis would not have been a factor in making my heart act up. But the murmur gave me little trouble. I gave up tennis and instead would take five-mile hikes. Everything was fine and dandy until I attained thirty-eight or nine. At that time I began to develop the characteristic pressure pains on the chest upon walking after a meal, or where it was upgrade, but found that by taking vitamin E I could do so without any trouble at all.

About twelve years later, or a year after I began to travel to Europe, I found that I had to increase the dose of vitamin E to keep the symptoms of over-activity in check. Looking back now I wonder whether the increased coffee drinking or crossing the ocean by airplane had anything to do with it. I cannot say.

65. Skipping Coffee Entirely

About two years ago I decided to cut out coffee to see if it would aid my heart condition. For six weeks I did not drink a single cup but soon found a severe worsening of my heart condition as expressed in chest pains upon exertion. I had no trouble in cutting out coffee, except that I seemed to lose my enthusiasm for work. It is rather strange, however, that at first I did not associate the return of my heart symptoms with the fact that I was not drinking coffee, but one bright day the possibility did occur to me and I began to drink it again. Within one day I became free of the unpleasant heart symptoms.

When I described my experience to a physician he told me that he recalled some medical researches done in Austria which indicated that when there was damage on the right side of the heart, coffee drinking was an absolute must to stimulate it. I did a little checking up myself in the medical literature and found the following statement in the *Deutsche Medizinische Wochenschrift* of August 25, 1950: "These investigations and the fact that caffeine dilates the coronary vessels and thus improves the metabolism of the myocardium suggest that there is no justification for interdicting either caffeine or coffee in patients with hypertension (high blood pressure)."

Another medical article says, "Coffee has the following definite pharmacological properties. It is a good stimulant of the central nervous system and of respiration, a fair diuretic (promoting urination), and coronary artery dilator and cardiac (heart) stimulant. . . . The toxic dose of caffeine for man is so large (over ten milligrams) that no human fatalities have ever been reported," (from *Aviation Medicine,* Pages 179, 185).

So coffee dilates the coronary vessels! This is probably what it was doing to me, and a good thing too!

About eight months ago I explained all this in an article in *Prevention* (January, 1954), and what a deluge of letters came in as a result! People told me they were amazed that an editor of a health magazine would drink coffee! Not one of them gave any scientific proof about what they were recommending. Most of them were flattering, indeed, saying how badly I was needed to raise the level of health of our country and that if I did not give up coffee drinking, they wouldn't guarantee how long I would live. This was a very profound experience for me—to think that all these well-meaning people were so concerned about my welfare, and I sincerely thank them, for they helped me.

I decided to cut out coffee again! I was feeling in wonderful condition. A year had gone by since my last tilt with old demon caffeine, and with this extra year of vitamin-taking and good nutrition under my belt, I figured, who knows, perhaps I could do it this time without a return of the heart symptoms. About two weeks afterwards my wife and I went to Europe again and before long the old chest pains returned upon exertion. But I would not give up. I decided to keep on with my program of no coffee, thinking that it would take time for my nervous system to build itself up. But

[176]

I found instead that it kept getting worse. But here is the most significant aspect of my experience—I found that without coffee my mind was not as active. Whereas on previous trips to Europe I had returned with piles of notes and written observations, this time I did not have one-fifth of the usual amount. I usually made on-the-spot notes, but when something interesting was observed or said I seemed to be too mentally sluggish to take my paper out of my pocket.

This reminds me of the experience of Herbert Spencer, the great philosopher who wrote: "I tried vegetarianism for three months and found I was obliged to destroy everything I wrote during that period because of a lack of meat." In my own case coffee seems to be my meat. But I persisted for a few weeks after I returned home, drinking no coffee. However, I soon had to hoist the white flag, because I was not only worried about my chest pains, but the quality and quantity of my writing was suffering. Immediately on resuming coffee drinking I was able to walk without pain symptoms and it became a pleasure to sit down to write. To me it is nothing short of miraculous.

66. Three Cups of Coffee a Day

Don't forget that the average person who has heart symptoms like mine would be taking digitalis and nitroglycerine and God knows what other drugs. For me, and for the rest of my life, it must be coffee, vitamin E, and all my other vitamins and minerals.

[177]

Louis Berman, M.D., in *Food and Character* (Houghton Mifflin, 1932), says that "caffeine and caffeine-like substances are the only ones definitely discovered to be brain stimulants and to be so employed the world over." I wonder if there have ever been any famous scientists, musicians, writers or philosophers of definite genius caliber who were not coffee drinkers. How about the vegetarian George Bernard Shaw? Did he drink coffee? I do know, however, that he took liver tablets, and they are definitely energy producers.

Regarding my own experience, I must state that I went back only to a three-cup-a-day basis and in connection with this reduction I discovered an interesting fact. When I consumed six cups of coffee a day there was always an intense craving for more, in between cups. I was always fighting off the desire to drink another cup, and could hardly wait for the time for the next one, which was an indication that the drug was in my blood, a condition similar to that which exists in the case of cigarette smokers. But when I began to drink coffee again I remembered all of the letters I had received from my readers and decided to fight any tendency to go above three cups a day.

Strangely, it required no struggle at all. I found that three cups a day gave me the effect I required without drugging the blood. I experienced no cravings in between cups. And I can thank my readers for being responsible for this reduction. A health magazine is for the purpose of educating its readers. In this case, however, the readers educated the editor.

I always drink my coffee black—no cream or sugar. In this respect I came across an interesting French medical research of experiments with injections of caffeine into rats which showed that the exciting effects of caffeine on the nerve centers are eliminated by an injection of sugar at the same time. In other words, there is a curious physiological antagonism between sugar and coffee. It was also concluded that the taking of sugar with coffee would greatly reduce the effect of caffeine on the heart. (*Comptes Rendus des Séances de Biologie,* Vol. 199, 1945, pp. 394-395.)

There is an angle to this coffee drinking problem that I must dwell on and it came to me as I was reading a medical article which showed that, in individuals on poor diets, drinking coffee could produce vitamin deficiencies, which means that this effect could not be brought about in people with good nutrition (*Archives of Biochemistry,* 1945, vol. 6. "Studies on the Nicotinic Acid Content of Coffee"). On the other hand a person who has an exceptionally good diet, including the taking of sufficient vitamins and minerals, can take a reasonable amount of coffee in his stride.

This reminds me of a piece of medical research which showed that painters who are exposed to lead can prevent themselves from getting lead poisoning by taking vitamin C. There is a terrific amount of evidence of other similar cases covering a variety of vitamins that can reduce or eliminate the effects of body poisons. This principle should be encouraging to those who cannot stop the coffee-drinking habit. But they should be sure to strengthen their bodies with the necessary nutritional augmentations as well as to get plenty of physical exercise.

67. Pulse, Blood Pressure and Coffee

A word of caution about coffee drinking. I would like to say that one should not drink his coffee too hot. In some susceptible individuals it may cause bleeding gums. Let it cool somewhat first. Also if you do drink coffee be sure that you do not make it in an aluminum utensil. Aluminum is a soft toxic metal and under the effect of heat some of it will get into the coffee. Dr. Arthur F. Coca in his book *Familial Non-reaginic Food Allergy* showed that coffee made in aluminum raised the pulses of some of his patients whereas if it was made in stainless steel or enamel it did not. Incidentally, I have checked the effect of most foods on my pulse. On the average, one half hour after eating each item of food my pulse would go up from three to twelve beats per minute, but in the case of coffee it does not even rise one point.

The experience with my blood pressure and coffee is also interesting. For the last four or five years my blood pressure has been pretty close to normal, but during the last period, when I was off coffee, a doctor examined me and said that I had high blood pressure. A few weeks ago, after taking coffee regularly, when I had it checked again it was back to a perfect figure. This, therefore, is an extremely assuring fact regarding coffee drinking in my own case. However, others have told me that coffee drinking raises their pulse and blood pressure so that it is a matter for individual consideration.

I would like to reproduce a letter, dated August 11, 1951, received from Theodora E. Ruther of Greenfield, Mass., which shows that coffee drinking helped another person: "Last fall I was having quite a lot of trouble with gas, sour stomach and heartburn and to relieve it I began taking an Allimin garlic tablet each morning after my breakfast. As long as I took them I got relief for the time being and got along through the winter very nicely. Then towards spring I stopped taking them and my former trouble returned again. Well, to make a long story short I had occasion to visit a brain specialist and in telling him my troubles I mentioned my stomach disorder. He suggested that I drink black coffee which I did of course, being willing to try anything that would put an end to my trouble. Now after three months of drinking black coffee I do not have any trouble at all from gas, belching, heartburn or sour stomach each morning. I also leave out sugar from my coffee which I have done for about 20 years."

In review let me say that I would not encourage children to get into the coffee drinking habit but that I would far rather see them drink coffee later on than get into the smoking or alcoholic drinking habit.

It is too bad that real thorough, scientific research has not been done on the subject. At least a thorough statistical poll should be taken showing the age of death, and the number of persons in each age bracket who are coffee drinkers. In the meantime, all about me are extremely old people who take coffee but in practically every such case you will find that these oldsters take it in moderation.

In conclusion may I say that God has given us

[181]

strong, rugged bodies which do not easily get out of commission. Give them reasonably good care and they will go with you nicely to the end of the line. I say reasonably good care. It is only one out of a million who can be perfect in every iota. I am sure that if I could cross-examine those who have previously written me advising the complete elimination of coffee, I would find other habits they have which are just as bad if not worse. It is the total score that counts, my friends.

It is not the function of a health editor to say to his readers, "Go out and sin," but he also cannot say to them, "Be superhuman." All I can say is that you should always try to be human, and as good as you possibly can be. But don't grow wings!

68. Evidence Against Coffee

We made a very significant observation in our research on the scientific proof of the harmfulness of coffee-drinking. From 1900 to 1915 medical and scientific journals were full of articles on experiments done. From 1915 to 1925 there were far fewer articles. From 1925 to 1945 the number declined still more. And from 1945 on there has been, practically speaking, little or no investigation of the effect of coffee on human health. We do not know what this may mean. Does it mean, perhaps, that medical men are discounting the facts discovered earlier and hence do not think it worth while to pursue the investigation further? Does it mean that new drugs, chemicals and poisons now demand so much time that we cannot spare time to investigate older substances? Or does it mean simply that physicians and researchers alike have decided that the fragrant brown beverage most of them drink all day long can't possibly need any further investigation?

69. Additional Evidence Against Coffee

As far back as 1746, a treatise was published on *Tobacco, Tea and Coffee* by Simon Pauli, an Italian writer. Pauli appears to be a writer of some substance, for his works were accepted widely among the learned of his day. We know there were many misconceptions about physiology in those days and of course present-day methods of investigation were not available. Yet it is startling that Pauli believes "it (coffee) is esteemed a great cooler (thirst quencher) for which reason it is drank by most, but if it is used to excess, it extinguishes the inclination to venery and induces sterility." He tells us further that in ancient times women of the East used coffee brewed extra strong as a purgative to prevent conception. Perhaps this is the reason why its use was forbidden to women for many centuries by the early caliphs. He advances the theory that coffee induces sterility because it gradually dries up the body's pro-creative powers on account of the large amount of sulfur it contains.

[183]

Later in our own country a writer on health, Dr. William Alexander Alcott, wrote that coffee is essentially and properly a medicine—a narcotic. He quotes authorities of that day (his book was published in 1844) as saying that coffee possesses nervine and astringent qualities, is suspected of producing palsies, has a powerful effect on the nervous system, a pernicious effect on the stomach and bowels, exhausts the sensibilities of the part on which it acts, induces weakness, produces debility, alters the gastric juice, disorders digestion and often produces convulsions and vertigo, feverish heat, anxiety, palpitations, tremblings, weakness of sight and predispositions to apoplexy.

He quotes Dr. Hahnemann, founder of homeopathic medicine, as saying that "coffee is strictly a medicinal substance. All medicines in strong doses have a disagreeable effect on the feelings of a healthy person." He also quotes Hahnemann as saying that coffee drinking produces the following diseases: nervous or sick headaches, toothache, darting pains in the body, spasms in the chest, stomach and abdomen, costiveness (constipation), erysipelas, disease of the liver, uterus and bones, inflammation of the eyes, difficulty in breathing and bowel affections. He compares the action of caffeine to that of arsenic, lead or prussic acid, asking "will anyone attempt to say that these substances are not poisonous because they poison slowly?"

Dr. Alcott is a cousin and associate of Amos Bronson Alcott, who was a famous educator and the father of Louisa May Alcott of *Little Women* fame.

70. It Is An Established Fact That Caffeine Is a Poison

Now perhaps these older writers may have jumped to conclusions when they laid down the unqualified statement that coffee was responsible for all the ills mentioned. Undoubtedly they did not use present-day laboratory methods to prove their statements. But they must have questioned their patients as to whether or not they used coffee and based conclusions on the answers. So while it does not follow that coffee-drinking was the sole and only cause of the symptoms their patients described, it does seem quite possible that coffee-drinking may have played a part in them. And it does seem significant that so much was written in times past about the possible harm of coffee-drinking. We do not find treatises attacking the use of apples, potatoes, carrots, bread or cheese. So we know, that, from way back, physicians have been concerned with the medicinal and narcotic aspects of coffee. And we cannot discount this concern as an old wives' tale.

We know that caffeine, the substance in coffee which apparently is responsible for its effects on the human body, is a powerful poison. A drop of caffeine injected into the skin of an animal will produce death within a few minutes. An infinitely small amount injected into

[185]

the brain will bring convulsions. The amount of caffeine in a cup of coffee is quite small. Yet we drink coffee because of the effect of the caffeine, just as we smoke because of the effect of the nicotine. Both are drugs, both are habit-forming. We uncovered some interesting accounts of headaches produced as "withdrawal symptoms" when coffee-drinking was abruptly stopped. We also know that efficiency of work performance decreases when a confirmed coffee-drinker stops taking his daily dose of coffee. These are symptoms typical of addiction. When any drug is taken away from a drug addict, he suffers "withdrawal symptoms."

71. Habitual Coffee-Drinking and Stomach Ulcers

What do some of the modern researchers have to say about the effect of coffee on the human body? There are two modern disorders that the general public usually associates with coffee drinking—ulcers and heart trouble. This may be mostly because physicians frequently forbid coffee to their heart and ulcer patients. There seems to be no doubt that coffee is bad for the ulcer patient, although we do not find any researcher who has proved that coffee actually produces ulcers in human beings. J. A. Roth and A. C. Ivy whose animal experiments on coffee are famous, tell us in *Gastroen-*

terology for November, 1948, that 1. Caffeine produces gastro-duodenal ulcers in animals to whom the drug is given in a beeswax container so that their stomachs are absorbing caffeine continually. 2. Caffeine moderately stimulates the flow of gastric juices. 3. Caffeine produces very definite changes in the blood vessels of animals which are similar to changes produced by prolonged resentment, hostility and anxiety. 4. As we know, one difficulty involved in ulcers is an excessive flow of hydrochloric acid into the stomach. Most peptic ulcer patients, say Drs. Roth and Ivy, respond to caffeine with a prolonged and sustained stimulation of the output of free hydrochloric acid. In other words, coffee causes more and more hydrochloric acid to pour into the stomach of the ulcer patient for quite a long time after the coffee has been taken. So, say these authors, although they cannot prove that caffeine causes ulcers, still it does seem that taking fairly large amounts of coffee may contribute to the development of ulcers and may aggravate the condition of an ulcer that exists already.

An investigation carried on at the University of Oklahoma by Vern H. Musick, M.D., Howard C. Hopps, M.D., Harry Avey, M.D., and Arthur A. Hellbaum, M.D., and reported in the *Southern Medical Journal* for August 1946 involved a total of 39 patients —10 of them with no symptoms of digestive tract trouble of any kind, 25 of them patients with duodenal ulcers and four patients with gastric ulcers. The researchers found that the flow of digestive juice is considerably increased in the normal person when caffeine comes into contact with the lining of the stomach. In the patient with duodenal ulcer the flow of digestive juice is "prolonged and excessive." Dr. Musick, in discussing the subject before a meeting of the Southern

[187]

Medical Association concluded, "I think it is all right for the normal person to drink caffeine-containing beverages but an ulcer patient or a patient who has a high secretory curve (that is, someone with a generally high level of hydrochloric acid in the stomach, which might predispose him to ulcers) should not drink coffee. He should not drink alcohol and by all means he should not drink black coffee the next morning after alcohol.

Now you will notice that, in all of these researches, caffeine was used—not coffee. This might lead someone to say "Well, of course straight caffeine is bad for you, but there is so little caffeine in coffee that surely coffee can't hurt me." On the same basis one could say there is so little nicotine in cigarettes, so little preservative in processed foods, so little arsenic on the outside of a sprayed apple, so little fluorine in fluoridated water, that there is no harm in taking any of these either. Once you begin to add up all these "small doses of poison" that you are taking every day, the sum total gets to be quite frightening.

Dr. R. Wood, M.A., B.M., B.Ch., B.Sc., writing in the *British Medical Journal* for August 7, 1948, tells us of experiments with cats in which he found that caffeine in the stomach has a powerful action on histamine, a substance which regulates gastric secretion. He also found that theobromine and theophylline (substances that occur in cocoa and tea) also have a similar action in some animals. "Our results support the Roth and Ivy conclusions," he says, "that ulcer patients should restrict their intake of beverages containing caffeine and also that it is desirable to limit their consumption of foods and drinks containing theobromine and theophylline."

[188]

72. Coffee, Heart Disorders and Blood Pressure

Concerning heart trouble and coffee-drinking, most nutritionists and books on health state that coffee has a definite effect on the heart and blood pressure. According to James S. McLester, M.D., in his book *Nutrition and Diet in Health and Disease* (W. B. Saunders, 1927) coffee raises the blood pressure slightly, slows and strengthens the heart, stimulates renal activity and prevents fatigue and depression. It also gives mild brain stimulation. He goes on to say that its excessive use is harmful, for stimulation and irritation are closely related. In cases of insomnia, cardiac irritability and rapid heart beat, even one cup a day will cause trouble when the heart is already irritated. More than one cup is especially harmful.

H. M. Marvin, M.D., in his book *You and Your Heart* (Random House, 1950) states that the effect of alcohol, tobacco and coffee all vary among different individuals. Some find that their heart beats faster after a few drinks of alcohol or cups of coffee. Others find that their hearts beat just a little faster, or not at all faster. He says that no one knows why this should be so. Perhaps some people develop a "tolerance" for coffee and others do not.

That word "tolerance" keeps recurring in all the literature about coffee. Our medical dictionary defines "tolerance" as "the ability of enduring the influence of a drug or poison, particularly when acquired by a continued use of the substance." It seems peculiar that the word should be used in speaking of coffee if indeed coffee has no harmful effects on the body. And, is it possible that those of us who suffer no apparent ill effects from coffee have simply accustomed ourselves to it over a period of time, so that we can throw off the ill effects?

Kathryn Horst, Rex E. Burton and Wm. Dodd Robinson, writing in *The Journal of Pharmacology and Experimental Therapeutics,* Volume 52, 1934, tell of an experience involving a number of young men whose blood pressure was tested before and after they began to drink coffee habitually. The maximum rise in blood pressure occurred during the first week they were drinking coffee. Later on, the article explains, a "tolerance" was developed, and the blood pressure remained at the same level.

When the coffee was withdrawn, the blood pressure returned to "normal." We don't know how you interpret this experiment, but to us it seems to show definitely that some substance in the coffee does have an unhealthful effect on the blood pressure. For those who can, after a time, build up a "tolerance" to this effect, the blood pressure does not go higher. But what of those who do not build up this tolerance? Might not coffee be a very important factor in continued high blood pressure which, of course, is one of the most widespread disorders in our country today?

73. Coffee Tars and Cancer

Does the use of coffee have any relation to cancer incidence? There is at least one researcher who believes that it does. We know well that certain kinds of tar produce cancer. Coal tar is cancer-producing. The tar from tobacco products produces cancer in laboratory animals. A. H. Roffo in an article published in *Boletin del Instituto de Medicina Experimental,* volume 15, 1939, describes obtaining tar from coffee. He found that this tar has the same physical characteristics as that obtained from tobacco. He treated laboratory animals with this tar and 73 per cent of them developed tumors which ended as cancerous growths. In a later experiment he fed coffee tar to rats in non-toxic doses. That is, they did not receive enough of the tar to make them ill at any one time, for he was trying to discover what the long-continued effect of the tar would be. Definite sores in the stomachs and digestive tracts soon became ulcers which eventually developed into cancers.

Roffo believes that it is the roasting of coffee that produces these tars. He also says that they are not soluble in water, so perhaps they are not present in coffee as we drink it. Still, in chemical tests such as spectography and fluorescence, the coffee tars show the same characteristic as coal tar. This is the only scientific evidence we could find of a possible relationship between coffee-drinking and cancer. It seems strange that no one has done any further investigating to find out, for instance, how much, if any, of the offending tar we drink in a cup of coffee. Or, perhaps, is the tar that ugly black scum that settles on the bottom of the coffee pot and is so hard to wash off, if the coffee has been standing for any length of time? Come to think of it, that black scum looks and acts very much like the black deposit on the bottom of a very dirty ash tray.

74. Does Coffee Affect Brain and Nerve Tissue?

The Department of Agriculture published a booklet in 1917 called *The Toxicity of Caffeine*. Their experiments involved animals. They tell us that the reaction of human beings and animals to caffeine may be quite different. Yet most scientific research these days (on chemicals, insecticides, cosmetics and so forth) is done with animals and it is taken for granted that any substance that shows up as poisonous to animals is quite likely to be not very good for men.

The authors tell us, too, that the effect of caffeine on individual animals is different in its intensity and the effect varies with the dose. On the same basis, undoubtedly some human beings are less resistant to poisons than others. William Salant and J. B. Rieger, authors of the booklet, tell us that only one rabbit in ten survived injected doses of caffeine. Those that survived generally succumbed to a second or third dose. The effect of caffeine on guinea pigs was even more drastic, although dogs and cats reacted differently. All showed symptoms of poisoning, which resembled poisoning from strychnine. It relation to its harmful action on tissues (chiefly brain and nerve tissue) caffeine is far more destructive than morphine. They conclude that the continued use of caffeine-containing beverages over a long period of time seems bound to be harmful.

Well, would you consider giving your family—children and old folks included—ever so small a dose of morphine every morning as part of breakfast, no matter how much they might like the taste? Keep in mind that caffeine showed up as being far more destructive than morphine.

This is the bulk of our evidence on the possible harm that may result from habitual, prolonged and excessive coffee drinking. It does not seem to us that someone who drinks one cup of coffee a day should go to a lot of trouble to give it up. But probably he will be the person who could give it up most easily. The person who is in danger from coffee, we believe, is the person who simply can't get along without it and who, if he stops and soberly counts up how many cups of coffee he has in any one day, may find that coffee is indeed a drug to him and that the habit of throwing off weariness and worry with a cup of coffee has brought him nothing but sorrow and ill health. These are the people who should be persuaded to give up coffee entirely.

If this should prove to be impossible, we have one last suggestion. According to our standards, we should eat and drink nothing that does not contribute in some way to nutrition. Any food or drink that contains neither vitamins, minerals, enzymes or protein should automatically be crossed off the list, for it is crowding out in our diets those beneficial protective foods we all need so desperately. If you must continue to drink coffee, then at least make certain that the rest of your diet is as healthful as possible. This means plenty of

[193]

fresh raw fruits and vegetables every day along with plenty of good meat, eggs, fish and nuts. This means only completely whole grain cereals. This means no food at all that contains white flour or white sugar in any form, even including chewing gum and soft drinks. This means taking food supplements: fish liver oil for vitamins A and D, brewer's yeast or desiccated liver for the B vitamins, rose hips for vitamin C and wheat germ oil for vitamin E.

75. About Tea

"In order to rightly estimate the advantages of tea, we must not look at its value abstractly, but on the influence it exercises on the country at large. We look at its use as one of the greatest counteractors of intemperance, for the man who enjoys his tea with his family is not a person who seeks the stimulus of the tavern, and in the lower classes the public house and the gin-shop. These are pitfalls purposely placed to entrap the footsteps of the unwary. Few are so heedless as to fall into a pit if exposed to their view; but the warmth of the fire, the brightness of the lights, the temporary excitement of the draught are as flowers strewn over the chasm beneath. We do not go as far as to say that good and cheap tea would in any decided manner remedy this evil. But we do say this, and every man who has bestowed a thought upon the subject will agree with us, that the man who enjoys a good cup of tea and can get it, with its necessary concomitants, fire and comfort, at home, will not be in much danger of turning out after the labors of the day to seek the poisonous excitement of the drinking house."

So said an anonymous writer in London in a little booklet called *The Tea Trade*, published in 1850. It seems that, not only in England but in other countries as well, tea has been introduced and promoted for the express purpose of luring wayward fathers of families away from stronger drinks. A Chinese legend tells us that tea was first used in China in 2737 B.C. However, it is first mentioned in Chinese literature in 350 A.D. Its use spread rapidly through China and Japan under the guidance of the Buddhist priests who were trying to combat intemperance. The United States at present consumes only about seven-tenths of a pound of tea per person annually, where the British use about 10 pounds.

76. How We Get Tea

The tree which produces tea looks a little like myrtle and blossoms like a wild rose. When the leaves are being picked, the end ones—that is, the newest and tenderest ones—are picked for high-grade tea. The next leaves down on the branch for the next grade of tea and so forth. In all about 3,200 leaves or "shoots" are necessary for one pound of tea. There are over 2,000 possible blends.

In processing black tea the leaves are "withered" with heat, then rolled and allowed to ferment. For the green tea, the leaves are withered in hot pans, then rolled and dried. Oolong tea is partially withered at ordinary temperatures before it is dried. The fermentation of black tea removes some of the tannin, so that a cup of black tea properly made contains less tannin than a cup of green tea.

It appears that the criterion for excellence in tea is the amount of caffeine contained in it, in relation to the amount of tannin. The aim seems to be to achieve a tea high in caffeine and low in tannin. It is suggested that the best way to do this is to infuse the tea only 5 or 6 minutes and then immediately pour it off the leaves. For making tea, the water should be freshly boiled, the water and tea put into a hot teapot, then the brew poured off into another hot teapot. And, of course, teapots should always be of crockery, glass or china, never metal.

Tea contains caffeine, tannin or tannic acid and essential oils. The caffeine is the stimulating element, the tannin gives tea its color and body and the oils give it flavor and aroma. Tea contains 2.5 to 5 per cent of caffeine and 7 to 14 per cent of tannin. The tannin in concentration has an unpleasant effect on the mucous membranes of the mouth and digestive tract, but in the concentration in which it appears in a cup of tea it is not believed to be harmful. It is, of course, the same substance used widely in medicine as an astringent and for skin diseases and burns.

77. Whether or Not You Should Drink Tea

In general, everything we say about caffeine in relation to health applies to tea as well as coffee, except that the caffeine content of tea is not so high. Then too, it appears that there are fewer people in this country in danger of becoming tea addicts. There are, of course, people who drink tea in quantity, people who simply cannot get along without their tea. These folks are caffeine addicts just as the coffee drinkers are.

There is one aspect of tea which should be mentioned, because of the recent controversy over water fluoridation. Tea, as we drink it, is extremely rich in fluorine. A government booklet tells us that cheap grades of tea may contain as much as 398.8 parts per million of fluorine. Many of our foods contain fluorine in its natural form, in combination with other food minerals. So far as we have been able to determine, this naturally occurring fluorine is not harmful, any more than naturally occurring iodine in foods is harmful, in spite of the fact that a concentration of purified iodine, not combined in a food product, is of course poisonous.

If fluorine is indeed powerful against tooth decay as the "experts" would have us believe, how does it happen that the English people, drinking such quantities of fluorine in their daily tea, do not have wonderful teeth? As a nation, the British people have notoriously bad teeth. So far as we know, the "experts" who are promoting fluoridation, have never explained these curious facts.

We would say, however, if the water in your locality is fluoridated, you would do well to stay away from tea because tea-drinking is bound to add considerably to your fluorine intake. And the fluorine in tea does not appear with other minerals as it does, for instance, in the case of bone meal. Bone meal provides the calcium necessary to neutralize the toxic effects of fluorine, according to W. J. McCormick, M.D., of Toronto, Canada.

[197]

So, if your local water supply is fluoridated and you still feel that you cannot get along without your tea, perhaps bone meal as a food supplement would be your best safety bet.

78. Seeds and Mental Power

April, 1956, *Prevention:*
Is there such a thing as a brain food? It used to be thought that fish was such a food. Nutritionists in discussing the phosphorus contained in fish refer to it as being a brain stimulant. But this idea has been more or less debunked. Let us, however, consider seeds as a food for the brain. Seeds will also satisfy the requirement for phosphorus. In fact, they contain ten or twenty times more phosphorus than fish. Seeds are truly a brain food.

It is known that animals fed raw grain seeds can perform much more work than those grazing pasture grass exclusively. This, of course, is work, not brain power, but let us look a little further.

I will quote G. A. Sutherland, M.D., in his *A System of Diet and Dietetics,* 1925: "Thus among the rodents, the stupid rabbit, unable to climb and with little prehensile power, has to be content with a bulky diet of comparatively innutritious herbs, while the more intelligent squirrel, a nimble climber and possessed of considerable prehensile power, is able to procure highly nutritious seeds and a considerable amount of animal food as well. The intelligence and nimbleness of rats, again, enable them to procure highly concentrated and palatable foods, and to place under contribution even those that man has stored for his own use."

Again, later on, this author states: "The frugivora, which include animals like the squirrel, the rat, and the monkey, consume vegetable food in its more concentrated forms, such as seeds and nuts. Being generally more intelligent than the herbivora, and gifted also with the inconsiderable prehensile powers, they are able to pick and choose their food more cleverly; and hence securing it in much more concentrated forms, they are provided with a much less bulky digestive system than the herbivora."

In the early primitive days of civilization, while man ate plants and fruit, a goodly part of his diet was in the form of seed which was consumed without any cooking, tampering or processing. In this regard Dr. James Empringham in his book *Intestinal Gardening for the Prolongation of Youth,* gives a remarkable instance of how food can sharpen the faculties of the human body. He says: "In the Pyrenean mountains, that separate France from Spain, there is the most interesting cave the writer has ever explored. At some remote time, masses of rock fell down, completely covering up the entrance to this natural, subterranean chamber, so that this marvelous museum of prehistoric art remained buried, according to geologists, for at least fifty thousand years, until rediscovered by accident some years ago.

"That the cavern had been the resort of human beings in former ages is evident from the rude drawings that still decorate the interior. These sketches consist, for the most part, of outlines of animals, long

[199]

extinct, which hitherto were known to science solely by the fossilized remains found in the Earth's rocky strata. The roof of this cave is embellished with representations of the midnight sky. But among familiar constellations, such as the Great Bear, there appear stars that can be seen by no person now living, except with the aid of a telescope.

"Now, inasmuch as the savages of that distant age had no knowledge of glass, and possessed no instrument for assisting the eye, these pictures seem to prove that the people of that far off time, had much stronger vision than men of today.

"Strange as it may seem, there is much evidence to prove that, not eye-sight only, but all of the senses of modern man—hearing, feeling, tasting and smelling—are less acute than the faculties possessed by our remote ancestors."

In biblical times a great deal of seed food was part of the daily dietary. Dill and cumin seeds were considered so important that tithes were paid with them. In his book *Jewish Magic and Superstition,* Rabbi Trachtenberg says that Baladur (anacardia) was a memory-strengthener. He advises further for strengthening of the memory, "Eat hazelnuts for nine days, beginning with 6 and adding 6 more each day; eat pepper seeds for nine days, beginning with one seed and doubling the dose until it reaches 256 seeds on the ninth day, and each time before you consume them, recite Deut. 33:8-11 and Psalm 119:9-16; grind cloves, long peppers, dates, ginger, galanga-root, and muscot nuts in equal quantities, beat them with olive oil into a paste, and eat a little every morning before breakfast."

The Romans, at the end of their gluttonous feasts, ate spice cakes flavored with aniseed. Seed cakes charged with a large variety of seeds were a standby of the Middle Ages. Vernon Quinn, in *Seeds—Their Place in Life and Legend,* describes an Englishman of Pepy's time commending seeds as "marvelously good for a melancholicke person, excellent fine for such as be of a cholericke nature even to free the sleep from monstrous nocturnal visions."

There seems to be some evidence of a dependence in olden days on eating seed to strengthen the mind, to free it of conditions brought about by dissipation, or to cheer it up generally. Our common sense should tell us that the mind is nourished by the food we eat, and that seed food, containing so much potent, living quality should be an excellent means of maintaining mental health.

Today there seems to be a noticeable deterioration in mental energies. With so much consumption of cola drinks, white hot dog rolls, ice cream, candies, etc., by our teenagers, is it any wonder that colleges are complaining of insufficient applicants for the more difficult courses of science, chemistry, etc.? Will there be enough technicians in the future to man the complicated Frankensteinian system of science that is being set up today? Researchers must be set going to re-evaluate all the factors of our nutrition insofar as it affects the operation of our minds as well as our bodies.

Is it possible that a body that is strengthened by consuming a certain portion of live seed food will be proof against cancer? Who knows? Nobody has researched it.

We once had an old parrot, about 90 per cent of whose diet was sunflower seed. And was he smart! He could sing a wonderful soprano, trilling in human fashion, without uttering a false note. When a knock came on the door he would always say "Come in!" That is intelligence! Many a cola-consuming teenager

[201]

today who hears a knock on the door is too lazy to say "Come in."

The value of seeds in furnishing human mental energy should be investigated.

79. Magnesium and the Teeth

IN THE February, 1962, issue of *Prevention* there began my series on magnesium that was to create somewhat of a sensation in the field of health. My interest in this mineral began about 15 years ago, in connection with my editorship of *Organic Gardening and Farming*. From time to time I would come across interesting facts about dolomite, a rock that contains a large percentage of magnesium. Ground as fine as talcum powder, it was plowed under as a soil amendment, or fertilizer.

Slowly I had accumulated a large file of data on the use of magnesium by people to improve their health in many ways. It seems to have been the forgotten mineral, and about 50 per cent of the American public was deficient in it, with some detriment to their health.

The first article in this series which I alluded to above showed that it was magnesium rather than calcium that prevented cavities in the teeth.

I will quote from my article:

Over a period of three years a magnesium compound (magnesium phosphate) was administered to a group of 200 patients ranging in age from 5 to 56, in whom it was noticed that there was a significant reduction in the number of cavities in the teeth. The following are details of 7 extracted teeth of persons who received the magnesium compound, all of whom had a great reduction in the incidence of caries. In these cases tooth extractions occurred, and these teeth were tested for their calcium and magnesium content, as follows:

CALCIUM	MAGNESIUM
4.73	.22
4.33	.13
3.65	.42
4.19	.49
4.35	.30
4.31	.10
3.50	.30
Average 4.15	.28

The following are the figures for the extracted teeth of persons who did not get the magnesium compound and who had more caries:

CALCIUM	MAGNESIUM
4.75	.03
4.60	.05
4.75	.19
4.70	.27
4.42	.08
4.13	.28
4.60	.14
4.50	.12
Average 4.55	.14

We can adduce several things from these figures. First, the magnesium from the magnesium compound taken by group 1 showed up to a certain extent in the teeth, and it is believed by the researchers that this magnesium gave the teeth a resistance of caries.

[203]

Secondly, it appears, according to this project, that calcium does not play a part in preventing caries, which is proven by the fact that the United States consumption of milk is very high, as is also its caries rate. Milk, a food very low in magnesium, is not a cavities preventer. But bone meal, which is very high in magnesium, is definitely a factor in preventing caries. Kelp also is a food supplement high in magnesium.

The researchers, evidently being aware of the world-wide fluoride controversy, went to the trouble of entering a statement in their paper to the effect that the magnesium compound they gave was fluoride-free.

Incidentally, only 7 examples were given of the teeth of persons who had received the magnesium compound because these were the only ones of the 200 cases that had had teeth extracted.

From 1962 to 1966 (August) not a letter was received by us questioning in any way the broad statement that it is magnesium, not calcium, that prevents cavities. But the fallacy is so well entrenched that it will be a long time before dentists and doctors are aware of the truth.

As I have observed it, the practice of medicine and dentistry today is rife with erroneous and fallacious beliefs.

80. High Magnesium in Egypt—Low Cancer

BACK IN 1939 when I ran a series of articles on cancer, in my *Fact Digest* magazine (discontinued in 1942), I became interested in magnesium as an aid to bodily health. I will quote from one of those articles, which will explain my interest:

Let us talk about the researches of Professor P. Schrumpf-Pierron, whose work is written up in the *Bulletin de l'Institut D'Egypte,* Vol. XIV, Feb. 15, 1932, and others. He talks about the rarity of cancer in Egypt where malignant cases are only about one tenth that of Europe. What is the cause? After exhaustive studies and research the Professor came to the conclusion that it was due to too much potassium and too little magnesium in the foods of Europeans. On the other hand in the soils of Egypt the conditions are reversed, that is, more magnesium in relation to the potassium.

There seems to be a definite relationship between magnesium and potash wherever it is found, whether in the soils, rocks or other places. Where there is an oversupply of potash there is always an undersupply of magnesium and vice versa. Schrumpf-Pierron studied the cancer statistics for France in relation to the rock structure underlying its soils. It worked most uncannily. Wherever he found an excess of potash there he discovered less magnesium and more human cancer cases. Wherever he observed a minimum of potash he found a maximum of magnesium and less cancer cases. This means that people who eat food raised in certain soils that obtain their nutriments from the rocks which underlie them get certain elements in their foods because of this. Such a condition would apply more to France than to the United States because in a country like France there would be more of a tendency to consume food near the point at which it is raised. But in the United States, with our more advanced industrial condition where even the poorer peoples eat winter vegetables raised in California, Florida, and elsewhere, and

[205]

a great deal of citrus foods and meats that are shipped long distances, local deficiencies and unbalancings of nutritional elements may tend to be corrected to a certain extent.

When Schrumpf-Pierron found that an excess of potassium in the rocks of a region tied in with an excess of cancer cases in that section, we should note that excess potassium means excess carbohydrates in plants grown there and therefore, reduced protein in the foods. Farmers should know that it is best, therefore, to use dolomitic limestone when they apply lime, because it is rich in magnesium and acts as a safety factor in relation to the potash in the soil.

At this time I would like to discuss my *bete noire*— milk drinking. Dr. S. Marcovitch, quoted above, says in the same article, "Milk with a low magnesium ratio, while an excellent food for the young, may be detrimental for adults."

Here is another reference: "Some component of milk interferes with the utilization of magnesium. R. H. Smith (in *BioClinical Journal* 67, 472, 1957) . . . recently undertook the elucidation of this phenomenon" (*Nutrition Reviews,* June, 1958).

In my files I find several proofs that good results in coronary cases can be obtained by the use of magnesium. Here is S. E. Browne, M.D., writing to *Lancet* (London, Dec. 9, 1961), who says that for the past 9 months he has injected a magnesium sulphate solution into patients with severe angina or a history of coronary thrombosis with excellent results on 5 patients with really severe angina.

Another piece of evidence is in an article in *Lancet* (Nov. 1, 1958) which says, "Recent work has suggested that magnesium may be related to atherosclerosis and ischaemic heart disease. It has been claimed that magnesium sulphate is of therapeutic value in myocardial infarction, while a high magnesium diet has prevented the development of atherosclerosis in rats." Not a word about potassium.

In the *British Medical Journal* (Jan. 23, 1960), an item contains the following: "Over 100 patients suffering from coronary heart disease . . . were treated with intramuscular [injected] magnesium sulphate with only one death, compared to their findings in the previous year when, of 196 cases admitted and treated with routine anticoagulants, 60 died."

81. More of My Magnesium Series

IN THE JULY, 1964, issue of *Prevention* the article on magnesium covered alcoholism. I will quote from it:

An article on magnesium in *Annals of Internal Medicine* (47: 956, 1957) in which alcoholism and magnesium are discussed contains the following summary: "A clinical syndrome characterized by muscle tremor, twitching and more bizarre movements, occasionally by convulsions and often by delirium, has been described and is considered to be a manifestation of magnesium deficiency. The evidences for this concept are the many similarities to experimental animal magnesium deficiency, the occurrence of low mean serum magnesium concentrations for a group of patients, a positive magnesium balance during treatment, and, finally, the frequently gratifying and sometimes dramatic response to therapy with magnesium salts."

An important statement in this article is that the taking of magnesium can lower the blood pressure. People with high blood pressure could perhaps try magnesium therapy, but only under the supervision of their physician.

A newspaper column by Dr. H. L. Herschensohn, in the *Arizona Republican,* some time in 1958 said: "For years, epsom salts was given to persons suffering from acute alcoholism. The good effect was partially due to its cathartic action, but it was also due to the fact that epsom salts, being magnesium sulphate, makes up for the deficiency of magnesium characteristic of alcoholism.

"In animal experiments, when the magnesium in the blood is decreased, tremors occur similar to delirium tremens . . . magnesium is an important part of every cell in the body. It is possible that its deficiency, even in non-alcoholics, may account for some ailments which are difficult to diagnose."

In the August issue the subject of magnesium and the teeth was discussed, but we have already discussed this.

In the September issue, magnesium's effect on cholesterol was discussed. I will quote part of it:

The authors state that coronary thrombosis (blood clots) is reported to be uncommon in Africans. In Johannesburg the disease is very rare among the Bantu. In one series of 352 post-mortems of Bantus over 50, only one death was found to be caused by a coronary thrombosis.

In another study of 523 post-mortems of non-Europeans, there was an incidence of 1.6 per cent of coronary thrombosis in the 41-60 age group. This contrasts with a figure of 12.8 per cent at the Massachusetts General Hospital.

[208]

The authors state, "Serum cholesterol levels are lower in the African native than in the European." But the cholesterol level in the newborn Bantu is the same as in European babies. Something happens after birth, to give the Bantu the advantage, as far as cholesterol is concerned. It probably is the diet, and the active physical life led by the natives.

In a study of 70 healthy South African Europeans the cholesterol level was 215. In the Bantus, of similar age and sex, it was only 174.

"In view of our striking results with magnesium sulphate therapy in coronary thrombosis, and the low cholesterol levels and low incidence of coronary occlusion in the Bantu, we decided to investigate the serum-magnesium level in European and Bantu groups, and to find out whether it was correlated with the serum-cholesterol level. . . . Serum-magnesium levels were determined on 47 normal Europeans and 53 normal Bantu (all 25-45 years)." The results were 1.92 for the Europeans and 2.11 for the Bantus. According to the investigators this .19 advantage of the Bantus' magnesium is "highly significant."

More magnesium serum studies were made and the authors summarized: "These results show (1) that the magnesium level is significantly higher in the non-European than in the European, and (2) that a definite correlation exists between serum-magnesium and serum-cholesterol levels. . . . Where the serum cholesterol content is low the magnesium content is significantly increased. . . . These findings suggest that the part played by magnesium in the diet and nutrition requires further study. The possible role of this element in cholesterol metabolism, and indirectly perhaps in atherogenesis (hardening of the arteries), has not been fully appreciated, studied, or recognized."

In the October, 1964, issue, it was shown that on the average, Americans are deficient in magnesium. I will give a short excerpt:

There can be no question that the United States public on the average is eating a diet deficient in magnesium. This is true because:

1. Magnesium in wheat is mainly in the wheat germ, but the general public favors white bread. Only 19 per cent of the total magnesium in the whole wheat remains in the white flour.

2. The average person drinks milk and eats cheese and butter in which there is very little magnesium.

3. Vegetables are rich in magnesium but the cooking water takes out more than 95 per cent of it!

Under date of June, 1964, the *American Journal of Clinical Nutrition* published a 50-page article by Mildred S. Seelig, M.D., entitled "The Requirement of Magnesium by the Normal Adult." This discussion points up serious deficiencies of magnesium in the nutrition and the bodies of American people.

In November, 1964, the subject was kidney stones and gallstones. In part it said:

We will now discuss the effect of magnesium on kidney stones. I will first quote from *Health Bulletin* (June 13, 1964) published by the Rodale Press:

"Magnesium oxide 'looks very promising' as a preventive of kidney stones, Dr. H. E. Sauberlich of the Army's Fitzsimons General Hospital in Denver told *Health Bulletin* this week. He said that results he has been getting with a 250-milligram tablet made from the same material used to manufacture fire bricks could spark a revaluation of the present methods of treating kidney stones.

"The new therapy is simply taking one capsule daily. Assisted by three researchers from the University of

Colorado Medical School, Dr. Sauberlich prescribed this capsule for a group of volunteer patients who had histories of passing kidney stones. After only a very short time on these pills, he pointed out, the patients had no more stones. That happened with each of the patients he has followed up for as long as two years, Sauberlich added. No side effects have been encountered.

"The odd part about the new therapy, which is strictly experimental and not conclusive, is that none of the researchers understands why or how magnesium prevents kidney stone formation. The only clue they have to go on is that a patient with this disorder 'for some unknown reason requires more magnesium than normal amounts.' Tracking down the reason and devising a test to discover those individuals who have this unusual requirement is the next step, Sauberlich said.

"A possible hint to the way the Denver researchers will attack the problem came when Dr. Sauberlich was asked whether a dietary deficiency was implicated in the kidney disorder. Although he stated that at present no such association exists, he was quick to point out that 'magnesium as a dietary requirement has not been adequately studied.' "

Further information on the above research was given in the *Medical Tribune* (June 3, 1964), which said, regarding Dr. Sauberlich's work:

"Therapy consisted of a single tablet of 420 mg. of magnesium oxide, which provided 250 mg. of magnesium ion, daily. Longest period of treatment to date is two years, and none of the 14 have passed urinary tract calculi while undergoing treatment, Dr. Sauberlich said.

"He detailed two cases of the magnesium therapy after other methods had failed. A 34-year-old man had passed a calculus about every other week for 11 years, but passed none while receiving therapy for six months. When the therapy was temporarily withdrawn, he began passing calculi within two weeks. Since returning to therapy he has been asymptomatic [without symptoms] for a year.

"A 38-year-old man had a 10-year history of weekly kidney stones. Magnesium therapy stopped this for 12 months, at the end of which the patient decided on his own to discontinue treatment. Calculi recurred within two weeks, and Dr. Sauberlich observed that he gladly resumed therapy, also on his own. He has been asymptomatic again for three months.

"Coinvestigators were G. E. Bunce, Ph.D., and Drs. C. A. Moore and O. C. Stonington, of Fitzsimons and the University of Colorado Medical School."

And in the December issue the subject was how to get enough magnesium. All the details are too complicated to be described here. So all I will say to you is to get some dolomite tablets in some health food source and take at least 6 a day. Thousands of *Prevention* readers have been taking it for several years with no harmful side-effects.

82. Prostatic Trouble

ONE OF THE pieces of work I have done which has fascinated me a great deal is acting as a compiler and observer in connection with the prostate gland. But first may I say that about 1945 I began to experience trouble in urinating. There was a burning sensation. This was the beginning of a prostate condition. To make matters worse, I experienced a pain at the end of the reproductive act.

But slowly over the years as I began to regulate my diet (beginning in 1950) and to take the various minerals, vitamins and lecithin, the situation came under complete control, and by 1955 it was entirely gone.

I wrote an article in *Prevention* about how important it was for prostatic cases to undergo the whole Prevention system and we later received some letters from readers who had cured prostate conditions by following the general idea of getting the whole body into good health.

I remember one case in which a man from Denver, Colorado, was in a hospital, to be operated on for the removal of his prostate gland the next morning. He had brought along some magazines. One of these was *Prevention* in which there was an article on the prostate. After he read it he told the doctor that he had changed his mind and that he was going home, which he did. By applying what he had read in *Prevention* he soon got his prostate into pretty good shape. On a trip to New York, this man later on stopped off to see me and to thank me for having published the article that saved his prostate.

I thought you might be interested in the particular article. It was in the May 1955 issue of *Prevention*.

Earlier articles mentioning the prostate gland and difficulties that may arise around it have brought in so many inquiries from *Prevention* readers that we did considerable research to uncover whatever else we could find that might be helpful for readers who want to avoid "prostate gland trouble" later on. We found precious little information. The prostate gland is removable. Because prostate trouble can be cured by an operation, little definitive research has apparently been done on what causes such trouble and what, aside from an operation, can be done to help.

If the prostate gland were not situated as it is, the enlargement that occurs so frequently in later years might go completely unnoticed. But for some mysterious reason this gland is located around the mouth of the bladder. So when it swells it cuts off the tube leading from the bladder and, since urine cannot flow freely as before, complications arise rapidly.

The prostate gland is an auxiliary sex gland, concerned with manufacturing the fluid in which the sperm cells float. Hence the removal of the gland results in sterility, even though generally it does not otherwise affect the sexual powers of the individual. In some cases it may. Until quite recently, removal of the prostate gland was a dangerous operation with a high mortality. In recent years less than 2 per cent of patients die of prostate gland operations. The time in the hospital has been cut to a minimum and in general, members of the medical profession urge removal of the gland when it is causing difficulty.

Since disorders of the prostate occur mostly in the years past middle age, it might seem likely that surgery mortality would be high because of the advanced age of the average patient. We have the word of John A. Taylor, M.D., of New York in the *Journal of the American Medical Association* for October 27, 1951, that prostatectomy (removal of the prostate gland) is not especially hazardous even for patients in their nineties. Since 1945, 41 operations have been done at St. Luke's Hospital on patients over eighty, and Dr. Taylor has performed 27 operations on his private patients over eighty. In one case the patient was 96 years old. Most of the patients had other diseases as well, the most common of these being hardening of the arteries and heart disease. There was a total mortality of 3.1 per cent among elderly patients which seems to indicate that the operation, as performed today, carries little risk.

What possible role does good nutrition play in preventing disorders of the prostate gland? The fat-soluble vitamin seems to be most concerned with the health of this gland, just as they are with the well-being of cells and tissues throughout the lining of the digestive and reproductive tracts. We know that a lack of vitamin A has a very definite reaction on these tissues. One of the earliest symptoms of vitamin A deficiency is a sloughing away of cells on the lining of the digestive, respiratory and reproductive tracts. Just as the tissues of nose and mouth may clearly indicate a vitamin A deficiency, so the delicate and sensitive tissues of the reproductive tract reflect any deficiency.

We know, too, that vitamin E plays an important part in the health of the reproductive tract. Many experiments with animals have shown that a deficiency in vitamin E will create all kinds of problems in sexual life, for both the male and the female. In animal experiments these difficulties can be speedily corrected by giving vitamin E. This is one reason why good animal feeds always contain ample vitamin E.

Wheat germ oil, too, is noticed for its effectiveness in preventing disorders of the sexual organs. It is given to both males and females in animal experiments and has proved itself of great value. It is believed that the natural hormones that occur in wheat germ oil are responsible for its powerful effect. It is made from the reproductive part of the wheat, of course, and carries with it all the substances that safeguard the reproductive processes of the grain.

Vitamin F (the unsaturated fatty acids) has been named by two researchers as curative of enlarged pros-

[215]

tate gland. To ensure that I get enough of this vitamin I take 3 capsules of lecithin a day.

James Pirie Hart and William LeGrande Cooper, M.D., of Los Angeles, California, conducted an experiment involving nineteen patients to whom they gave unsaturated fatty acids. No other treatment was given. Writing about this experience in a pamphlet published by the Lee Foundation for Nutritional Research, Milwaukee, Wisconsin, these investigators give their results as follows:

1. All cases showed a lessening of residual urine—that is, urine remaining trapped in the bladder. In 12 of the 19 cases there was no residual urine at the end of the treatment.

2. For 13 of the 19 patients, the treatments ended their getting up at night to urinate.

3. There was a decrease in fatigue and leg pains and an increase in sexual libido in all patients.

4. Cystitis or bladder inflammation cleared up as the residual urine disappeared.

5. Dribbling was eliminated in 18 of the 19 cases.

6. The force of the urinary stream was increased.

7. In all cases the size of the prostate gland was rapidly reduced.

Dr. Sieve's theory in general is that vitamins and hormones (the substances produced by the body's glands) work together to create health. Infection, emotional upsets and mechanical interference with food intake prevent a proper nutritional state. In studying 200 cases, Dr. Sieve found that infection was one of the main causes of nutritional decline in 60 per cent of the cases. Among men the most prevalent source of infection was the prostate gland. Along with the infection went nutritional deficiency and disorders of the glands and hormones. All three had to be cleared up in order to get the patient back into a healthy state.

Dr. Sieve made a careful study of 100 patients who suffered from prostate trouble. The age range was from 15 to 75 years, with the majority in the 43-63 age group. In 70 per cent of these the stage at which it would have been necessary to operate was prevented and no operation was necessary. Dr. Sieve's treatment, by his own admission, is purely preventive. He does not guarantee anything in the way of cures for patients with advanced cases. Instead he suggests that treatment should be started in the thirties, especially in those men who have a history of recurring infections. The younger the patient, the easier it is to correct his nutritional state, hence the infection, and hence the condition of the prostate.

The first patient he describes was 20 years old and suffered from headaches, lack of appetite and pain in his legs. He also had acne, brittle, ridged fingernails and other indications that all was not well nutritionally speaking. Dr. Sieve prescribed a full and well-balanced diet, along with vitamin supplements containing vitamins A, C, D and E and the vitamin B complex. In addition, he was given another preparation containing vitamin B.

And, in case there might be difficulty in assimilation, vitamin injections were given once a week. The patient was also given by mouth and by injection various hormone substances that his condition indicated he needed. In addition a course of prostatic massage was given. Four years later the young man was quite well. He was still taking the vitamin preparations, and Dr. Sieve said he hopes the youth realized their importance enough to go on taking them the rest of his life. He also stated that he could predict that this patient would never suffer from prostate enlargement, barring acute infection.

The second case was 35 years old, a man who complained of fatigue and extreme sluggishness as well as distress in his digestive tract resulting in gas, vomiting and abdominal pain. There were many other symptoms indicating wrong diet for a period of years. And the prostate was "boggy." In addition to the vitamins A, B, C, D and E in large amounts, this patient was given a capsule containing the fat-soluble chlorophyll substance from alfalfa, buckwheat and soybean (did this possibly contain the precious vitamin F?). Furthermore, he was given vitamin injections and gland medication. He had prostate massage once a week. And his prescribed diet was well balanced.

Twelve months later he showed great improvement in many directions. He had not noticed any stomach distress for more than eight months. He had lost 12½ pounds of excess weight. He had not been absent from work for a single day in seven months. The prostate gland was much smaller and no possibly dangerous nodules were to be found in it. For five years he continued to improve. Dr. Sieve comments that "a good . . . clue to the type of case in which prolonged infection can be anticipated is for example the individual who gives a history of having had severe acne at puberty."

He reminds us further that these cases of nutritional deficiency he is describing are not "full blown, classic textbook cases," but the findings all add up to "subclinical nutritional deficiency." That means just enough deficiency to bring about countless ills, such as acne, prostate enlargement, fatigue, headaches and so forth, but not enough deficiency to result in scurvy or pellagra or one of the other vitamin deficiency diseases. This is

the condition we talk about so much in *Prevention*—
this dragging, listless, tired state of health most of us
have, which could, with proper nutrition, be changed
to vital, glowing health.

The third patient Dr. Sieve treated was 55 and had
been warned by a number of specialists that an operation on his prostate was absolutely necessary. His com-
plaints were dribbling and frequent urination at night.
He had also suffered an attack of coronary thrombosis.
As Dr. Sieve examined him he noted many symptoms
of vitamin deficiency in nails, tongue, skin, etc.

His prescription was similar to those mentioned before—large doses and injections of all the vitamins and
treatment for glands. The prostate was massaged once
a week. Five months later the patient looked and
sounded like a new man—free from headaches, no pain
in his heart, better sleep and loss of all symptoms of
the prostate difficulty. At this time he was also given
the tablets made from the soybeans, alfalfa and buckwheat. At eight months even greater improvement was
shown and, says Dr. Sieve, the patient looked twenty
years younger.

You will notice that Dr. Sieve did not give his patients just one or two vitamins—they got them all, and
in large quantity, in addition to a good, well-balanced
diet. By a good, well-balanced diet we mean a diet high
in protein (meat, fish, eggs) with little or no food made
from white sugar and white flour products, a diet that
includes plenty of fresh fruits and vegetables and nothing that is refined, processed, degerminated or chemicalized. In addition, get your extra vitamins as Dr.
Sieve's patients did: fish liver oils for vitamins A and
D, brewer's yeast or desiccated liver for the B vitamins,
rose hips for vitamin C and, perhaps most important

of all, wheat germ oil, vitamin E and the unsaturated fatty acids, otherwise known as vitamin F.

Another case was that of a personal friend of mine who also saved himself from a prostate operation by following the whole Prevention system. Here is another cure, described in a letter from a chiropractor, R.F.M., who writes us:

"A recent issue of *Prevention* carried an article on the beneficial results of including vitamin F in the daily diet, also reference to the research done by the Lee Nutritional Research Laboratory in treating hypertrophy of the prostate gland. I have had some trouble along that line with my prostate gland for the past few years, and various kinds of treatment have not proved successful.

"I sent for the brochure from the Lee Foundation and read it carefully. The result they obtained with control groups, suffering with prostatic disorder, was almost amazing in its simplicity, and I decided to follow the method they used in the addition of vitamin F to my diet. My improvement was noticeable within five days. It was no longer necessary for me to go to the bathroom at night. The flow of urine was stronger, bladder pressure was relieved and dribbling ceased. I am including vitamin F in my diet, and intend to continue."

A reader who relieved a prostate condition by giving up a food to which he was apparently allergic is Mr. Jon Assenat of Charleroi, Pennsylvania. He writes, "I am nearing 70 and enjoying very good health. I was troubled with prostate one year, then I read in *Prevention* about cutting out orange juice. I had been taking it daily, but decided to stop. Since then I have never had trouble with getting up nights."

Prevention shuns citrus fruits because of their acid

content, which is too strong an acid for the body to handle. It can lead to all kinds of trouble, but I never thought it could be responsible for a prostate condition. Still, if its effect is to reduce the general health of the body, it might affect any gland or organ which happens to be in a weakened condition for some other reason.

In 1958 there began a pleasant correspondence between Dr. W. Devrient of Berlin and myself. He was a reader of *Prevention* and wrote me that he was curing patients of prostatic trouble by having them eat pumpkin seeds.

He had written an article in *Heilkunde Heilwege* in 1959 from which I will quote passages:

"At the age of 50 and over, more than 60 per cent of all men have this trouble, over 60 this increases to 80 per cent.

"One can note that there is repeated mention (in botanic medical sources) of pumpkin seeds as a vermifuge [to expel worms], but in only two cases is their efficacy as a medication in the preventive treatment of prostatic hypertrophy [enlargement] spoken of."

But evidently there were doctors before Devrient who used pumpkin seeds in cases of prostatic trouble.

Hugo Schulz, the eminent pharmacologist, mentions pumpkin seeds in only three lines of his "Lectures on the Effects and Usage of German Medical Plants" (*Vorlesungen uber Wirkung und Anwendung der deutschen Arzneipflanzen,* Leipzig, 1929). Only the plain people knew of the open secret of pumpkin seeds, a secret which was handed down from father to son for countless generations without any ado. No matter whether it was the Hungarian gypsy, the mountain-dwelling Bulgarian, the Anatolian Turk, the Ukrainian or the Transylvanian German—they all knew that pumpkin seeds preserve the prostate gland and thereby also male

[221]

potency. In these countries people eat pumpkin seeds the way they eat sunflower seeds in Russia: as an inexhaustible source of vigor offered by nature.

"Investigations by Dr. G. Klein at the Vienna University revealed the noteworthy fact that in Transylvania prostatic hypertrophy is almost unknown. Painstaking researches resulted in the disclosure that the people there have a special liking for pumpkin seeds. A physician from the Szekler group in the Transylvanian mountains confirmed this connection as an ancient healing method among the people. Dr. Bela Pater, of Klausenburg, later published these associations and his own experiences in the journal 'Healing and Seasoning-Plants' (*Heil- und Gewurzpflanzen,* 12, 18, 1929).

"My assertion of the androgen-hormonal influence of pumpkin seeds is based on the positive judgment of old-time doctors, but also no less on my own personal observations throughout the years. This plant has scientifically determined effects on intermediary metabolism and diuresis, (excessive urination) but these latter are of secondary importance in relation to its regenerative, invigorative and vitalizing influences. There is involved herein a native plant hormone, which affects our own hormone production in part by substitution, in part by direct proliferation (production of new growth). Anyone who has studied this influence among peasant peoples has been again and again astonished over the effect of this plant in putting off the advent of old age. My own personal observations in the course of the last 8 years, however, have been decisive for me. At my own age of 70 years I am well able to be satisfied with the condition of my own prostate, on the basis of daily ingestion of pumpkin seeds, and with that of my health in general. This beneficial result can also be found among city patients who are prudent enough to eat pumpkin seeds every day and throughout their life. But one must continue proving this to the city-dweller. The peasants of the Balkans and of Eastern Europe knew of the healing effect of these seeds already from their forefathers.

"After painstaking study I came to the realization that the pumpkin seed is able (1) to cure the first stage of prostatic hypertrophy (excessive growth) and (2) to improve the second stage by converting it back to the first stage, to say nothing of its preventive influence that is factually attested. Its manner of influence is so profound that a subjective improvement can often be observed even in the third stage. Thus, it can be made completely believable that active ingredients are present in the pumpkin seed that are able to eliminate the primary condition of swelling of the prostate and to the extent even that a favorable preventive influence can be exerted on cancerous degeneration."

Now here comes my role as a compiler. In the *Journal of the Maine Medical Association* (March, 1958), Doctors Henry Feinblatt and Julian Gant attacked prostate disease by a nutritional method.

A word should be said here about cancer of the prostate. For some unknown reason this gland is extremely susceptible to malignancy. When prostatic difficulties do occur it is wise, therefore, to make certain through a medical examination by your doctor that no cancer is present, before embarking on a system of self-cure. Sometimes surgery is the only recourse in such cases.

If the prostate swelling is simply a benign condition of enlargement, then the findings of Doctors Feinblatt and Gant, mentioned above, should be of great interest and help. As I said, the discovery of this treatment was a happy accident. It happened this way: Dr. Gant and

[223]

a colleague were treating a group of allergic patients with a mixture of three amino acids (components of protein)—glycine, alanine and glutamic acid. One of the patients thus treated volunteered the information that his urinary symptoms had disappeared while he took the amino acid mixture. This led to a trial of the same compound on nonallergic patients with urinary symptoms. Patients with enlarged prostates and associated urinary symptoms experienced prompt and rather spectacular relief. They remained free of the symptoms while taking the compound, but soon after discontinuing the medication, the symptoms returned.

In other words, the cure was obtained with the three amino acids—glycine, alanine, and glutamic acid, which are proteins, or nutritional substances.

The thought then occurred to me: Is it possible that pumpkin seeds contain large amounts of these three amino acids? This proved to be the case when we sent some to a commercial testing laboratory. It was a thrilling finding.

Sunflower seeds can be obtained from health food sources—a variety has been developed which has no shell and can be eaten with no trouble.

Here is more compiling: One of the reasons why pumpkin seeds are specific for the health of the prostate is their high content of zinc. We had some pumpkin seeds tested in a commercial laboratory and they were found to contain from 40 to 50 parts per million of zinc, which is a sizeable amount for this mineral.

T. A. Mawson and M. I. Fisher, two scientists of Canada's Chalk River Atomic Project, made an exhaustive study, in both animals and humans, of healthy and cancerous prostate glands to determine the difference in their mineral content. Reporting their results in the *Canadian Journal of Medical Sciences* (Vol. 30,

[224]

pp. 336-339), they found that zinc is stored in very high quantity in the healthy prostate gland and in the sperm-nourishing seminal fluid secreted by the prostate. More zinc, they found, goes into the prostate gland than into any other human tissue. More important, "There was evidence of a decreased zinc content in glands containing malignant tissue." These two Canadian scientists did not pursue their work far enough to look for reasons, but they were convinced there was a definite connection between the amount of zinc in the system and the health of the prostate.

It has been found that the semen itself is extremely rich in zinc. Three researchers, George R. Prout, M.D., Michael Sierp, M.D., and Willet F. Whitmore, M.D., who performed experiments with radioactive zinc and wrote about them in the *Journal of the American Medical Association* for April 11, 1959, conclude their article on zinc and the prostate with this paragraph: "Sperm are richer in zinc than any human tissue studied, yet the testis is relatively poor in this element. From this observation alone, it would seem that zinc is related to spermatic physiology. It is conceivable that the prostate acts as nothing more than a purveyor and receptacle for zinc until ejaculation occurs and at this time zinc is incorporated in the sperm in perhaps essential capacity. Certainly, under the conditions of the experiments, the unfailing appearance of Zn 65 [radioactive zinc] in prostatic fluid and the prostate suggests that prostatic fluid without zinc would no longer be prostatic fluid."

[225]

83. Magnesium and the Prostate

THERE IS A remarkable book published in French, called *Equilibre Mineral et Santé* (Mineral Equilibrium and Health), by Dr. Joseph Favier (Librairie le Francois, Paris). While the title indicates that it deals with minerals, the actual fact is that it deals mainly and specifically with the mineral magnesium—the miracle mineral. The book shows how valuable magnesium is as a medicament for many diseases, but its chapter on magnesium's effect on the prostate should be discussed in this symposium on the prostate.

Dr. Favier gives a Dr. Stora credit for being the first to discover magnesium chloride as an effective agent in treating urinary troubles of prostatic origin. He informed the Medical Academy of France of it, on March 18, 1930. Eight days later, Dr. Pierre Delbet submitted a report showing the same results with magnesium chloride.

When Dr. Stora spoke about his results to Favier, the author of the book we are discussing, Favier began to make inquiries among his physician friends. He found that they were all taking magnesium chloride. To his surprise he found that 4 out of 5 of them had been disturbed by difficulties in urinating, especially at night. And all of them, after taking magnesium tablets, found that their nocturnal urinating troubles diminished or disappeared.

[226]

Another doctor, Chevassu, gave him other interesting data about 12 prostatic cases whom he had treated with magnesium tablets. Ten of them were cured. One disappeared, and he does not know what the result was with him. The one that was not cured was left with nothing more than nightly urinatings. The interesting thing is that the general physical condition of all these patients improved. There is something about magnesium that is healthful for the body.

Dr. Chevassu speaks of his Case No. 4, a 77-year-old prostate patient who suffered a crisis of complete retentions of urine. He had to be probed in order to urinate. His prostate was very much enlarged. Probes were carried on three times a day up to November 24, and hot clysters (enemas) were administered. The first spontaneous urinating took place on November 25; the probes were cut off on December 7. On December 10, the patient urinated five times a night and he had a large residue.

The magnesium treatment started on December 14, the dosage being 4 tablets (2 g. 40), and went on until February 21, 1930. The nightly urinatings fell from five to three, and the residue dropped to 20 grams.

The patient, having recovered his strength and feeling very well, believing he was cured, discontinued the treatment. Urinating frequency increased and three days later, on February 24, the residue had gone up to 126 grams. The magnesium treatment was resumed, the urinating frequency curtailed, and on March 21, the patient informed the doctor that he urinates only two to three times per night.

Regarding patient 13, who had been a case of complete retention of urine: he was sent to the hospital in order to have an operation of the prostate performed— that is, to have his prostate removed. But Dr. Chevassu felt that the operation in his case would be too dangerous. He was therefore given the magnesium chloride tablets. Spontaneous urination occurred, and the patient left the hospital without the operation. From then on he had no difficulty or pain with his urinations. Thereafter the patient used to come to the hospital regularly, merely as a friendly visitor to show his gratitude to the doctor. He was, of course, taking magnesium tablets after he left the hospital.

Doctor Favier ends the chapter by saying that among the men who have been taking magnesium chloride tablets for many years none to his knowledge has suffered from prostatic trouble.

As far as *Prevention* is concerned, its policy is against the use of drugs, except in an emergency. In a situation where prostatic trouble has established itself, it would be wise to take the magnesium chloride tablets, but in a case where a cure has been obtained, or when any person wants to prevent this disease from taking hold, it is better to take the magnesium, minus the chloride, to get it in a more natural form.

At this point I would like to discuss another physician's experience with a magnesium drug, which I read about in 1952 in *The Archives for Pediatrics* for July of that year, entitled "Light Magnesium Carbonate in the Treatment of Acute Glomerular Nephritis," by C. L. Thenebe, M.D., of West Hartford, Connecticut. Glomerular nephritis is a form of kidney inflammation affecting the glomeruli of the kidneys and we had better stop there or you will get all mixed up in capillary loops, renal corpuscles and such, which isn't important when we're interested in the prostate. All you have to know is that nephritis is a form of kidney trouble, and let the doctors take care of the rest.

It seems that the usual practice in treating this form

of kidney trouble is to use magnesium sulphate which, by another name, is known, as epsom salts. The sulphates from my knowledge are bad actors and are implicated in the causation of cancer. Dr. Thenebe found magnesium sulphate to be nauseating to his kidney patients, so he changed over to magnesium carbonate. In magnesium carbonate, the latter fraction is quite innocuous. In fact, on the average about 40 per cent of the contents of plants is carbon. Dr. Thenebe used the magnesium carbonate on eight patients, and said: "Comparably, magnesium carbonate tastes much better (than magnesium sulphate) and is not at all nauseating. It is harmless in large doses." He obtained his magnesium carbonate from the Merck Drug Company.

What I would like to suggest is that since magnesium carbonate is much safer than the magnesium chloride we have been discussing under Dr. Favier's account of the treatment of the prostate, that it be tried instead of the magnesium chloride. Perhaps in emergency cases the treatment can start with the chloride form, and change over to the carbonate when the condition has alleviated itself.

I want to pause here and take credit for determining that dolomite is a good source of magnesium, in the form of magnesium carbonate. As a result, the health food industry has made it available to the public and today thousands upon thousands of persons are taking it with wonderful results. I take 9 tablets daily—3 at each meal.

No doubt you have heard of the Dolomites, a range of mountains in the Alps. Dolomite rock contains from 30-50 per cent magnesium. These rocks are known as dolomitic limestones, and they contain also large amounts of calcium.

There is medical evidence that if the general public

[229]

took dolomite tablets every day, it could add from five to ten years to the life span.

So—for a healthy prostate, be sure you have a high-protein diet of healthful foods (no sugar, bread, citrus, etc.), pumpkin seeds, dolomite tablets, and an hour's walk every day.

Here is a typical letter, one of dozens we have received in which people have described being helped regarding their prostate:

Dear Sir:

I have had prostate trouble for over 17 years. I had all the standard treatments, but none helped, except temporarily. Then on the first of March, 1965, I was operated on for an obstruction at the neck of the bladder and knots on the prostate gland. It helped lots, to relieve the pressure on my bladder. I still had the high pus count in my urine, also in my prostate fluid. I went to the doctor every other week for a massage of the prostate to keep down the pus count. I still had bad lower back pain. I went to a chiropractor 4 times a week for 3 weeks, then 2 times a month, still had backache. I had for 2 or 3 years taken some small pills that cost almost 85¢ each, per day for pus. Then I received your magazine, read your part on magnesium and the prostate, and started to take dolomite tablets, 10 per day. After about 4 weeks, no massage, my pus count dropped from 40 per whatever part they use to 9 to same part. I took no other drugs. To me that is worth crowing about and one of the best parts is my backaches have gone. I don't get up at nights anymore. Thanks to my good Lord.

Yours truly,
James R. Williams
Dublin, Georgia

84. More on Mastication

IN THE PAST I have stated that there are four factors determining the question of how much chewing of food there should be. *One*—the width of the esophagus; *two*—the occlusion of the teeth; *three*—the rate of flow of the saliva; and *four*—the amount of taste buds in the tongue. Now I have found a *fifth*—whether the saliva contains a certain enzyme, and how much of it it contains. The enzyme, called ptyalin, helps to break starch into a form of sugar that the body can absorb.

But it is our nervous system that controls our saliva. When food is placed in the mouth, certain nerve endings are stimulated and cause certain glands to produce saliva immediately. Therefore if we have a healthy condition of nerves and salivary glands, and if we are in proper general health so that sufficient ptyalin is produced, then much of the process of oral digestion is accomplished in quicker time than if those conditions are not present.

So, in some cases there will have to be more mastication than in others.

Another factor: if you are a 100 per cent Preventionite, if you go all the way, and don't eat bread, cakes, etc., there will be less of a problem because this type of grain food needs more mastication in the mouth. For example, if you eat a dry cracker, you will have to chew it until it turns to liquid. As far as meats are concerned, they don't require much deglutition, if you'll permit a fancy word.

[231]

But don't gulp meats down as a dog does, for it poses another problem. In the *Journal of the American Medical Association* (Oct. 12, 1963), cases are described of sudden deaths caused by food becoming blocked on the way down, shutting off the air passage. A case is described of a woman who gulped down a large piece of filet mignon, which became stuck in the pharynx and killed her. The death was first diagnosed as a "coronary." In the stomach were found large pieces of meat with no evidence of mastication. In this case the woman had ill-fitting upper and lower dentures.

Thus we see an application of item 2 above; malocclusion of the teeth. Dentures are not necessarily present—sometimes there is very poor occlusion of the natural teeth, and in such cases more time must be taken to grind up the food in the mouth.

85. Reducing Diet

It is about time we spoke about methods of reducing weight. There are hundreds of them, and many of them are worthy. I have used 10 to 20 of them, but here is my latest thinking on the subject, which seems to be working for me at present.

First and foremost is a dependence upon extra vitamins and minerals to protect you, in the first few weeks especially. As weight comes down, the body seems to temporarily lose some of its resistance to disease. That is why, in times gone by, some Hollywood actresses died so young. They allowed their weight to come down fast without the added protection of extra vitamins. But in the Prevention system generally, we are well protected in regard to the taking of vitamins.

2. The complete elimination of all wheat and rye products, and it must be quite complete, including breakfast cereals, spaghetti, etc. Bread is about the most fattening food there is.

3. No potatoes in the two or three months until you get down to a maintenance level, then potatoes in moderation. The starch of potatoes is more easily and quickly absorbed than bread starch. Wheat or rye bread in any form? Never!

4. No sugar—either white or brown. Raw sugar, in moderation, when on a maintenance diet later. Fruit, but not to excess. No candies, soft drinks, cakes, etc.

5. No factory-made foods! This leaves fresh non-processed meats, fresh fish, two eggs a day, fresh fruits and vegetables.

6. Be sure to add the protective seed foods, sunflower and pumpkin. These are extremely potent in nutrition and very helpful in keeping up the resistance of the body when pounds are coming off.

7. Vegetables—get a good array of all kinds and colors, not overlooking the leafy kind. Eat as many of them raw as you can. Corn on the cob in moderation is permitted, as well as brown rice.

8. Be sure to walk briskly at least an hour a day. In many cases, this really brings the weight down, especially if indulged in on very hot days. You must perspire.

Now how does it work out? Here is my breakfast: Two eggs, four or five medium-sized prunes (no sugar added) covered with wheat germ flakes, sunflower and pumpkin seeds in an amount that fits in the small part of the palm when you contract it, a tablespoon of a mixture of cold pressed oils (I use olive, corn, safflower

[233]

and sesame) and a drink of some kind (no milk). As far as the two other meals are concerned, one of them consists merely of raw fruits, raw vegetables and a drink. The amount? Don't stuff yourself. I include lettuce, radishes, raw peas, an apple or figs, asparagus, etc.—not all at one meal, of course. Your scale will tell you if you are overdoing it.

86. Third Meal

Remember, no soups ever, if you wish to lose weight.

A fairly good meat portion—such as steak, liver, roast beef, chicken—should be included. I have found steak and roast beef more fattening than chicken and veal. Add a cooked vegetable, and some raw vegetables in moderation. You can't go away hungry from this meal. You must eat enough.

It is best to eat the meat meal at noon time, if possible. It has time to be worked on before you go to bed.

After supper—only if you feel you must have it—eat a piece of fruit. If you need more than that, add a few raw vegetables.

No added salt is to be either cooked with food or taken at the table. Water should be drunk whenever you crave it, once a day with a dash of grape juice in it.

Here is a dish that will brighten up a dull reducing regimen: little corn griddle cakes:

Dissolve ½ cup of corn meal in 1/3 cup of cold water. To this add 1/3 cup of boiling water. Then beat in one egg or two if desired. It is optional also if you wish to grate an onion and put it in. Stir the batter and let it stand for half an hour, keeping the batter warm.

[234]

Then spread in small flat cakes on a griddle. It is just simply delicious and can make up for a lack of bread. But eat these in moderation!

Be sure to divide up your daily vitamin intake into three portions—one at each meal!

I have found it very helpful to keep a daily chart with my weight before and after each meal. It shows you when you are overeating. This may not be as easy, but is more fun, than watching the stock market.

So here you have my plan. I hope it works for you as it does for me.

EXTRA NOTE: A friend advises me of a plan I suggested to him many years ago, which took 40 pounds off for him: nothing but chicken, fresh fish, eggs, raw vegetables and very little fruit.

87. My Error

Eggs are my favorite food. They are the finest form of protein, superior to meat, and should be eaten by everyone, including heart cases. Don't worry about their cholesterol content, so long as you cut out other fatty foods such as butter, cream, ice cream, etc. The other day I decided to take my eggs raw, the yolk only, minus the white. Egg white contains a toxic substance called avidin, which is rendered innocuous by heat. In the past when I ate the whole raw egg, including the white, after a few days a dull feeling developed in my head. Years ago, when I went on a diet of the raw egg yolk only, after a few weeks I caught a cold.

I decided to try again. I worked out a very delicious dish—the raw egg yolk thoroughly mixed in apple sauce, sprinkled with wheat germ flakes . . . delicious! In two weeks, down I came like clockwork with a cold, something I never get anymore. And this in spite of massive doses of vitamin C as soon as the first sniffle came. Evidently there is something valuable for me in the egg white. This ought to be a lesson to some people who think that everything they eat should be raw.

On the other hand, this may not affect other persons as it did me.

Reducing: Years ago when I went on a weight reduction program, after I would lose about ten pounds I would get constipated. This no longer happens, probably because I eat no bread.

In the old days when I reduced, my general bodily resistance went down, and I would catch a cold more easily. Today this does not happen because I take so much vitamin A and C. In fact, my tremendous vitamin and mineral intake is an insurance against the untoward effects of poundage loss.

Years ago, when Jean Harlow, the movie star, died on account of severe weight losses in a reducing program, she might have survived had she been taking vitamins.

A few years ago when I reduced from about 175 to 162, I found the latter weight a sort of threshold figure. I use this word in a special meaning. Below this figure I began to experience a comfortable feeling. I would walk with greater ease or pleasure.

I figure that at this weight figure of 162 there is a proper distribution of fat throughout the body. Above this weight there is more fat, and it begins to get into the artery walls. This is sheer speculation.

MY OWN TECHNIQUE OF
EATING FOR HEALTH
INDEX

PAGE

[237]

PAGE

—L—

—M—

—N—

—O—

INDEX